PCOS

*Naturopathic Approach and
Plant-based Recipes*

Olivia Stein

Page intentionally left blank

Table of Contents

Introduction

I would like to commence this book with the following phrases: ***YOU ARE NOT ALONE!*** and ***PCOS IS TREATABLE!***

That is right! Whether you have already been diagnosed, or you are currently suffering from PCOS symptoms and have not been diagnosed yet, it is absolutely necessary to know that YOU ARE NOT ALONE! I know how you might feel! It can be quite confusing, and overwhelming at the beginning, and even after, when there isn't enough information provided for how to deal with it and you desperately start looking for a solution. The variety of books and research you read makes you feel frustrated and powerless, as that is just tons of information, and none of it can serve as a practical guide in your journey.

PCOS IS TREATABLE! Even though there is not any cure accessible for this condition, PCOS is still treatable. There is vague advice available such as: avoid stress, improve your sleeping patterns, change your lifestyle... Yet, it does not help that much. Who does not need to eat healthier, sleep better or avoid stress?

Ok, maybe some more than others, but still, knowing that, will it help you to fight against PCOS? Certainly it does not! Where to start off and how?

And that is why I felt the urge to create this book and I am so passionate about it. This book has been created with the solemn purpose to be used as a guide in taking your first steps towards PCOS recovery, reestablish hormonal balance and boost your immunity. I am not a doctor, but I am confident as this book is a product of years of research and practical experience. It will be of great value for you and will serve you as a manual in moments when you are not sure how to deal with the polycystic ovarian syndrome and how to get through this struggle.

According to dr. Priyanka over 70% of women's infertility issues arise due to PCOS and it affects 5-10% of women in the reproductive period. Its percentage depends on the woman's age. But beside being the most common endocrine female disorder and beside the continuous research, there is still lack of information about PCOS. It can be quite different for everyone and it depends on the situation and the immunity level of the individual. As a consequence, the doctors often have insufficient information (unless they are specialized for treating PCOS)and very often the condition remains undiagnosed and unmanaged.

I remember how shocked I was at the beginning when I found out that there are different types of PCOS and that one might suffer from PCOS without having the symptom of polycystic ovaries. Yes, even though the name PCOS implies that the ovarian cysts are central, the polycystic ovaries are not always part of PCOS.

Over the years, as I got to learn more about it, I realized that every aspect matters, and taking a holistic approach can be the answer for treating PCOS. Modern medicine still does not pay enough attention to the fact that body and mind are interconnected and taking a holistic approach can restore the symptoms of PCOS.

However, the positive outcome has been noticed for a variety of female conditions as a result of this approach.

Integrative medicine is quite an appropriate answer for PCOS, as the polycystic syndrome as a condition is slightly different from the others, due to the fact that it is a lifelong condition. The first signs of PCOS within your hormones are present from your childhood. Soon after, it evolves in a condition that affects the entire female body and can bring drastic changes to a woman's life. While it is a common belief that it is an infertility condition, actually it is not. It is an endocrine condition that impacts the reproductive system, mental and emotional state of being, metabolism, the immune system and the cardiovascular system. It affects the whole body and hence we can not expect to treat just one symptom or just one part of our body and to expect results. Everything needs to be taken into consideration. It's not that we need to just focus on that particular part of the body, but also on our entire lives and external factors, as PCOS is significantly impacted by the environment, stress, nutrition, activity ect. That is why it is important to increase people's awareness that PCOS is much more than anovulation and infertility.

Thank you for trusting me by buying this book and I congratulate you on deciding to take the first step by improving your life and fighting against PCOS.

CHAPTER 1: Understanding PCOS

The very fact that you decided to read this book means that you are already familiar with what will be discussed in this chapter. To me personally, at the beginning everything was so overwhelming, and the initial confusion seemed to be always present. Just after I started conducting in-depth research and understanding the different aspects of PCOS, it began to make more sense and I realized how PCOS is connected to our mindset, well being and environment.

PCOS is the abbreviation used for polycystic ovary syndrome, that is also called Stein–Leventhal syndrome or hyperandrogenic anovulation, due to the elevated presence of the male hormones, so-called androgens, which influences the release of an egg from the follicle, and as consequence it leads to ovulation issues and infertility. It is a hormonal disorder, and in most cases, women grow plenty of small cysts on the ovaries.

It is not a birth defect. The polycystic ovary syndrome is a result of a combination of environmental and genetic features. Moreover, obesity and lack of physical activities are some of the risk factors for this condition.

The common symptoms include: menstrual disorders, (irregular menstrual cycles or no period at all), difficulty becoming pregnant, excessive hair growth, gain weight, especially in the central area due to the insulin resistance, oily skin, acne etc.

The syndrome was firstly noted in 1721 in Italy, and initially was described by the American gynecologists Stein and Leventhal: "Young married peasant women, moderately obese and infertile, with two larger than normal ovaries, bumpy, shiny and whitish, just like pigeon eggs" (Vallisheri, 1721). Later, they further elaborated their research with regards to PCOS, and in 1935 PCOS was described in detail in their paper presented at the Central Association of Obstetrician and Gynecologists.

The Polycystic ovary syndrome is a heterogeneous condition that usually affects one of five women who are in their reproductive age. It is considered to be one of the most common factors that cause female infertility, and just in the US it affects 6% to 10% of women who are in their reproductive period. That equals to around 5 million of women.

The percentage slightly differs in the various countries. In India it is estimated that 10% of the women suffer from PCOS, and studies showed that in the UK, Spain, Greece and Australia around 6% to 9% of women are affected by PCOS. According to the World Health Organization, in 2012, on a global level, PCOS affected 116 million women, that is equal to 3.4%.

The syndrome can be quite stressful and frustrating for women. Besides causing pregnancy issues, it also increases the possibility for other diseases, such as: high blood pressure, insulin resistance, type II diabetes, dyslipidemia, sleep apnea etc.

There is no treatment available for this disorder. Still, as I mentioned, taking a holistic approach and implementing a significant lifestyle change, can remarkably keep all symptoms under control, including infertility.

PCOS and the Ancient hunter gatherer communities

So where does PCOS come from? Is it genetic? Is it caused by the unhealthy lifestyle and processed food we consume? What I found particularly appealing is that the polycystic ovarian syndrome is not typical for the countries where the obesity rate is higher. Hence, obesity can not be the main reason for PCOS.

Doctors still haven't provided answers about what causes PCOS, but evidently it is somehow related to genetics, and is provoked by a mixture of environmental factors and genetic predisposition. It is a genetic disease that is transferred from mother to daughter. So women that have precedents of PCOS in their family history have higher possibilities to suffer from the syndrome.

A new article by Fertility and Sterility suggests that the polycystic ovarian syndrome is an ancient genetic disease, and the PCOS symptoms as acne, increased abdominal fat, irregular menstrual cycles and infertility were noted in women over thousands of years ago. When I read this theory for the first time, I found it particularly compelling.

Back in the ancient times, the ones having metabolisms that could store fat and safe energy were considered to have had definite survival benefits, and this is typical for women suffering from

PCOS. They tend to carry these metabolic advantages and conserve the energy, which is of a great benefit in periods of low food supply. Furthermore, as a consequence of the reduced fertility, women with PCOS often had only one young child, and hence were at a survival advantage due to the greater resources for them and their family.

Usually, the fertility rate is lower amongst women with polycystic ovarian syndrome at all BMI - Body Mass Index levels. Still, compared to modern times, in ancient civilizations, women were more physically active and there was less of a food supply. Therefore, usually women with PCOS did not suffer from obesity problems, and even at times when there was lack of food, they were having normal levels of fertility due to the decrease in the Body Mass Index that in those times would reach the normal level. On the contrary, the BMI of the women who did not suffer from PCOS would considerably reach much lower levels thus making them predisposed to subfertility.

This indicates the importance of obtaining a healthy BMI in cases of PCOS and that the syndrome actually causes subfertility-delay in conceiving rather than infertility.

Another important fact to be taken into consideration is that men also carry PCOS genes. They also possess these metabolic survival advantages, even though they do not experience subfertility. The PCOS genetic variations are further passed from males to their offspring allowing the genes to persist for thousands of years.

Nowadays, the BMI levels usually tend to elevate as a consequence of the modern western diet and lifestyle, thus leading the effects on reproduction of PCOS to be intensified in comparison to those in the ancient times. It should be highlighted that the increased BMI is not the cause of the polycystic ovarian syndrome, but surely it is the reason for decreased fertility levels. Furthermore, patients suffering from high levels of insulin resistance which is supported by the western diet, would need to put extra efforts with an appropriate diet, supplements, and lifestyle change, in order to reach insulin balance in the body.

The misconceptions of PCOS

PCOS for sure is one of the most misinterpreted issues nowadays. Getting the medical diagnosis of polycystic ovarian syndrome, especially at the beginning, leads to a misconception that can put an extra weight on your shoulders that you do not need it!

One of most common myth for PCOS is that there is only one type of polycystic ovary syndrome. They slightly differ one from another, though what is surprising is that you might asymptomatically suffer from PCOS. I know it might be shocking and confusing, as it was for me, but yes, it is true!

The second misconception is that one symptom can be sufficient to get the diagnosis. PCOS is a group of symptoms so if you feel frustrated because you have one of the symptoms and your doctor still can not diagnose PCOS, it is because one symptom is just not enough for PCOS to be identified and treated. As said, PCOS can be diagnosed but you might not have polycystic ovaries, and also the opposite is possible: you might have polycystic ovaries and not have PCOS. The polycystic ovary syndrome can not be diagnosed with a simple test that shows if you have or do not have PCOS.

Also having excessive facial hair and/or acne is not enough for PCOS to be diagnosed. Women from various backgrounds and ethnicities would notice differences in the presence of facial hair.

Same refers to the acne that is not caused just because of PCOS and can have different causes, such as genetics, diet, hormonal changes during the puberty period etc.

The third misconception is related to one of the most painful topics for a lot of women: weight. Although women identified with PCOS are more likely to be overweight, the relation between weight gaining and PCOS is still not understandable.

Although, often women diagnosed with PCOS have problems losing weight, research conducted with relations to diet habits and behavioral changes, reported that women with or without polycystic ovary disorder can lose the same mass of weight.

Misconception number four: The polycystic ovary syndrome is a rare condition! As mentioned, about 5 million women in the US, in the period of reproduction, suffer from PCOS, which puts PCOS on top of the most common endocrine hormonal condition for women in the reproductive age.

Moreover, this number refers to women that have already been accurately diagnosed. Though PCOS often remains not identified, and according to the PCOS condition, this equals millions of women that are not identified with PCOS and unaware about their condition. This disorder makes around 70% of the cases and it is the cause of infertility issues that directly affects women who have ovulation difficulties.

The fifth misconception is that women suffering from PCOS cannot conceive a child. However, this is not the case with all women suffering from PCOS. The ovulation is the issue that provokes infertility, but it can be regulated with medications or various fertility treatments, as in vitro fertilization, and lifestyle changes.

Moreover, if you are not trying to get pregnant, and you do not use contraception pills because you have been diagnosed with PCOS, do not think you are safe. Although for sure it is more difficult to get pregnant in case you suffer from PCOS, still is possible, so there is a need to use the contraception pill in case you are not trying to conceive.

Types of PCOS

PCOS is treated as a single disorder and can look equal for everyone, and in spite of the fact that there is no official division, most of the doctors recognize four different types of the polycystic ovary disorder:

- insulin-resistance polycystic ovary condition;

- hidden cause PCOS;
- pill induced PCOS;
- inflammatory type of polycystic ovary syndrome.

Hence, depending on the type, a lot of the symptoms might overlap, but still some can be quite different.

Insulin resistance PCOS

The insulin resistance PCOS is the most common type of this condition. Hair growth in certain areas, hair loss and gaining weight are the typical symptoms for the insulin resistance type of PCOS.

With insulin resistance PCOS, the insulin does not respond to the sugar and stops performing its own role, i.e. to take out the sugar from the blood circulation. As a consequence, high levels of glucose and sugar are noticed in the blood. Other organs as the pancreas are also affected, as it tries to help reduce the sugar. The increased insulin affects the production of sex hormones and the ovaries produce more testosterone. Also, if you gain weight it might be the result of insulin resistant type of PCOS as the insulin inclines towards fat storage.

Smoking, trans fat, sugar and environmental pollution can be the cause for this type of PCOS.

Be careful with the sugar intake. Small amounts of sugar is fine, but as all things taken in excessive quantities have negative effects, sugar as well will significantly contribute towards worsening the insulin resistance.

In order to check if you have this type of PCOS, consult your doctor about testing the levels of glucose and insulin in your body. Being insulin resistant can significantly contribute to developing diabetes. Treating this type of PCOS is often a slow process and it usually takes between six and nine months in order to see the first improvements.

Post-pill PCOS

The post-pill PCOS is the second type that is most commonly identified and is usually diagnosed after women stop using the birth control pill. The birth control pills suppress ovulation, so usually, when women stop taking the pill, and they don't ovulate even months or years after the effects of the pill is completed, it can be a sign for pill induced PCOS. In case you had regular menstrual cycles before taking the pills and this is not the case after you stopped with the pill, be sure to visit and consult your gynecologist.

If you have experienced irregular menstrual periods also before taking the pill it might be that you suffered from the PCOS condition even before deciding to take the pill, but you were not diagnosed.

In case of post-pill polycystic ovary syndrome, the level of androgen and the level of LH is also increased. But, the levels of LH and FSH can be low as well, though what you need to pay attention to is the ratio of LH to FSH.

Hidden – cause PCOS

The hidden cause PCOS sometimes is referred to as an environmental type of PCOS.

It is one of the simplest types of polycystic ovarian condition as usually the ovulation is affected by stress, certain food choices, thyroid issues, poor gut health, lack of vitamin D, iodine or zinc.

The hidden cause type of PCOS probably is the one that can be speedily treated once the cause for it is identified and addressed, therefore the recovery process can take around 3 to 4 months. With proper lifestyle changes and a suitable diet this type can be simply treated.

Still, be careful to not treat it by yourself and test different methods, but always consult with your doctor.

Inflammatory type of PCOS

The inflammatory type of PCOS does not cause the typical symptoms of PCOS as gaining weight. As the name shows, what you will feel is inflammation in the body, manifested with headaches, joint pain, digestive problems, infections, skin issues as psoriasis or eczema. It can be caused by diverse factors, as stress, chronic viruses, food intolerances as gluten.

You can test the level of inflammation in your body with a test called hsCRP - high sensitivity C-reactive protein.

In case you suffer from an inflammatory type of polycystic ovary condition, pay attention to your diet, and avoid inflammatory foods, such as wheat, dairy products and sugar. Moreover, it is important to be careful about your lifestyle and avoid stress and toxins such as pesticides. The magnesium intake can help since it contains anti-inflammatory effects.

Also in this situation the recovery is a longer process and can take up to nine months.

Some of the experts also recognize a fifth type of PCOS known as **adrenal PCOS**, and in this case most probably you were not identified with any of the previous types of the syndrome, you have regular ovulation and normal level of testosterone, but you have increased level of adrenal androgens as dehydroepiandrosterone sulfate (DHEAS).

According to Doctor Lara Briden, who recognizes four types of PCOS: insulin-resistant, post-pill, inflammatory and adrenal PCOS, you can recognize your type by answering a simple survey.

You have been diagnosed with PCOS and you suffer from insulin resistance? Then you have insulin-resistance PCOS.

You do not suffer from insulin resistance, but you had normal menstrual cycles before taking the pill? This is the case of post pill PCOS.

You did not have normal menstrual cycles even before taking the pill? You have signs of chronic inflammation? If yes, you suffer from inflammatory PCOS.

If no, you need to check if DHEAS is the only androgen. If yes, in this case it is the adrenal PCOS.

I advise you to be more aware of the different types of PCOS and deeply research them as this is why some natural remedies may work for some women and for others not. Although women's experiences suffering from PCOS can be related, still there are quite a bit of differences among them.

Moreover, plenty of studies need to be definitely conducted for the various types of PCOS, as the official division still does not exist. And while some doctors can identify the type of PCOS, others are not able to do so.

In order to treat PCOS, it is of vital importance to treat the causes for it, and in case you are not satisfied with your doctor, make decisions on time, and choose another doctor that can guide you in the recovery process.

PCOS Symptoms

The first symptoms of PCOS can be noted in different phases. Often it happens when women get their first menstrual period, though it can happen when women cannot conceive.

The woman might not have any of the typical PCOS symptoms such as acne, weight gain and excessive hair growth or loss and might be misdiagnosed by her gynecologist as having an inexplicable infertility. Skinny patients that do not have the typical symptoms also can suffer from the polycystic ovary syndrome.

The Rotterdam Criteria set in 1990 during the National Institute of Health (NIH) conference established that women with PCOS have the following diagnosable conditions: an excess production of androgen (hyperandrogenism), ovulatory dysfunction (oligoovulation) and in 2003 the third criteria has been added and includes the multiple ovarian cysts or polycystic ovaries. The Rotterdam Criteria are applied by numerous researchers and medical experts, even though they are not based on evidence treatment guidance, but rather on expert meetings. Still, the Rotterdam criteria is the core of various clinical research and leading studies.

PCOS diagnosis can be confirmed if at least two of the three criteria are fulfilled:

- Long menstrual cycles or delayed ovulation;
- Hyperandrogenism;
- Polycystic Ovaries on Ultrasound.

Irregular menstrual cycle

Both, amenorrhea, a condition when you do not have menstrual cycles at all for three or more months, or oligomenorrhea, a situation when you have an irregular menstrual period, usually from four to nine times per year can be caused by the polycystic ovary syndrome.

The main reason why women with PCOS have irregular menstrual cycles is the hormonal imbalance. Each month your ovaries launch follicles in order to be fertilized. Though, due to the increased levels of androgens, the follicle does not get released by the ovaries, and remains inside of them. Hence, the ovulation is blocked and the follicle that is inside the ovaries can be seen also on the ultrasound. This symptom can vary: some women might have regular menstrual periods, others might have their periods each 30 to 40 days, while in other cases, women might not have menstrual periods at all.

Fatigue

Fatigue is an overall feeling of lack of energy and extreme exhaustion. It can take a great deal of your daily routines as you will feel as if you haven't had a good rest for a long time, in constant need to grab some sugar bites, and will constantly experience low energy. The afternoon energy drops, muscle weakness, poor concentration, difficulty to wake up in the morning and deal with the day, as well as stress situations are common side effects if you are experiencing fatigue.

Hair growth

The aforementioned androgens can also lead to excess hair growth in parts of the body where hair growth is typical for the male bodies. This symptom is known as hirsutism. Up to 90% of women that suffer from hirsutism have the polycystic ovarian syndrome, that also provokes further stress, as the hair can be coarse and present a challenge to remove it.

Pregnancy difficulties

Various factors can be the reason why women with PCOS have difficulty in conceiving or might need longer time to conceive. One of them is the irregular ovulation, so there is a struggle for the fertile window to be detected and there are few fertile periods annually. Another reason is the decreased egg quality as a result of the hormonal changes in the ovaries and the inflammation in the body. But, on the other side, women suffering from PCOS have an ample amount of egg cells, so usually it is just a matter of time for conceiving especially with the right treatment.

Acne

The acne can be caused by the increased levels of the testosterone. The polycystic ovary syndrome might be just one of the reasons for the acne. The dead skin cells, bacteria, oily skin, as well as stress and using comedogenic cosmetic products, also might be the cause of acne.

Apart from the acne, you might notice skin tags or dark patches, known as acanthosis nigricans, that might leave the impression that your skin is dirty but it can not be washed off even with hard scrubbing. The velvety discoloration of the skin is caused by the insulin resistance, and can be improved once the insulin resistance is reversed.

Gain weight

Fast gaining of weight can be an indication for PCOS. This is due to the insulin which usually helps the sugar from the food to be converted into energy, but in case of insulin resistance the sugar is built up in the blood circulation. The insulin also stimulates appetite and might make you feel hungrier. Intense cravings are typical for women who are insulin resistant, and can lead to creating bad eating habits and hence to weight gain.

The hormonal imbalance also contributes towards weight increase, as the hormones: leptin, ghrelin and cholecystokinin, which regulate the appetite might be dysfunctional for women suffering from PCOS and hence stimulate hunger as well.

Moreover, the increase of male hormones leads to weight gain in the zones where men usually gain weight, as is the central part or the abdomen. The abdominal fat is one of the most dangerous types of fat, as it is connected to higher risks of heart diseases and other various health issues, such as type II diabetes, sleep apnea, high cholesterol, high blood pressure.

Moreover, losing weight becomes more difficult so more than 50% of women suffering from polycystic ovary syndrome also suffer from obesity.

Male-pattern baldness

The polycystic ovarian syndrome also can cause hair loss as a consequence of the presence of the androgens, especially due to the presence of the Dihydrotestosterone within the scalp, which damages the hair follicles. For women suffering from this condition hair loss is often behind the hairline, right in the frontal area, but it can also be noticed all over the head.

Beside PCOS, also other conditions, such as ferritin and thyroid dysfunction can cause hair loss.

Ovarian Cysts

Due to its name, polycystic ovarian syndrome, PCOS indicates that the polycystic ovaries are central. Still, the ovarian cysts are an important sign, but not always present in cases of PCOS, that leads to a lot of women remaining undiagnosed. The cysts are actually partially evolved follicles. This usually happens to younger women, while the elder ones might not experience this as much.

Fatty Liver

Fatty liver, also known as NAFLD – Non-alcoholic Fatty Liver Disease can arise as a consequence of insulin resistance of the polycystic ovarian syndrome which leads the food energy, particularly the carbohydrates, to be stored as fat inside the livers. Fatty liver can be reversed, but if left untreated it might develop into serious conditions.

If you have fatty liver, it is important to take the necessary steps to reverse the insulin resistance.

Sleep apnea

The sleep apnea is a common symptom for many women that suffer from PCOS. They do not get enough sleep, and hence they experience daytime fatigue and tiredness. The sleep apnea can cause heart disease, mood changes, obesity and high blood pressure. Studies have shown that women with polycystic ovarian syndrome are the most insulin resistant and risk to develop obstructive sleep apnea.

Depression and Anxiety

Mood changes are common for women who suffer from PCOS as a result of the hormonal imbalances and the other stressful symptoms of it, such as acne, weight gain, infertility, hirsutism and irregular menstrual periods.Also,cortisol level fluctuations are related to anxiety and depression. The journal Human Reproduction confirmed that women with PCOS constantly have had increased levels of emotional distress.

Required laboratory tests

There are various conditions that can be related to the above symptoms, and getting comprehensive laboratory tests is one of the first steps that will help your doctor to diagnose whether or not you suffer from PCOS. All women that undergo fertility treatment, have acne, hirsutism, abdominal fat, or long menstrual cycle, no matter if they have gained weight or not, should do regular check ups of various PCOS symptoms. We will revise the top 10 most important tests for PCOS. I consider it important to get familiar with the language in order to be able to speak for your health and be well informed before making a decision.

Please be aware that some of the tests are recommended to be conducted on specific cycle days.

1. **Follicle Stimulating Hormone (FSH) and Luteinizing Hormone (LH)**

The Follicle Stimulating Hormone and the Luteinizing Hormone are two very important hormones secreted from the pituitary gland, which is a small master gland that controls the hormonal system. In case you have PCOS it is important to control the levels of FSH and LH as these hormones send messages to the ovaries telling them to release progesterone and estrogen, and hence, to prepare an egg for ovulation. The Follicle Stimulating Hormone has a role during the first part of the cycle when assists to grow the egg, while the Luteinizing Hormone gets involved a bit later and provokes the ovulation process. These two hormones react together, and their ratio is particularly important.

Usually the level of the Luteinizing hormone would be half of the Follicle Stimulating Hormone, or in some cases they will be on the same level. In case of PCOS, the ratio of LH:FSH will be reversed and increased, and the level of LH will be doubled or tripled of the level of the FSH.

Besides the ratio, the levels of these two hormones are important as well. If they are above 10 iu/L, it might be a sign that you are near perimenopause, or that the egg quality needs to be increased.

2. **Fasting Insulin and Glucose Levels**

Lot of patients that suffer from PCOS suffer as well from insulin resistance, which increases the testosterone production in the body, that is inflammatory and thus makes weight loss challenging and is associated with chronic illnesses. If you are insulin resistant it means that the cells in your body do not react to the presented insulin.

The insulin is responsible for bringing glucose in our bodies. But measuring just the levels of glucose is not enough without measuring the insulin resistance. Women can even have low glucose level, but suffer from insulin resistance. How is that possible?

Although insulin resistance is an alarm for diabetes, it is not diabetes. The diabetes might develop a few years after the insulin resistance. So you might have a normal level of the sugar in the blood and be highly insulin resistant.

Both metabolic indicators need to be checked and their ratio calculated. Doctors usually aim to see the glucose fasting levels under 5.0 mmol/L and a fasting insulin level below 50 pmol/L. Their ratio, which is called HOMA-IR, needs to be below 1.0.

The most sensitive exam is the insulin-glucose challenge test which takes 4 hours to be completed. This test can identify the insulin resistance at the most early phases, and hence can be an indicator of the PCOS treatments to start much earlier than normally.

3. Cortisol

Cortisol is a stress hormone that regulates most of the body functions. It impacts the metabolism, the immune system and the female hormones.

Usually the level of cortisol is increased in the morning, and then it decreases as the day passes by, to reach its lowest level in the evening when we start to feel asleep.

The cortisol test usually is done in the morning around 6-8 am and one of the best cortisol tests is 4 point salivary measurement, which estimates the involvement of this hormone in our daily routine. The normal level is 250 – 850 nmol/L. Low cortisol is an indication for congenital adrenal hyperplasia, a syndrome that imitates PCOS. But, women with PCOS usually have increased levels of cortisol which can affect the ovarian functions.

4. DHEA-S

The DHEA hormone is secreted by the adrenal glands and is placed on the top of the kidneys.

It is a direct indication for the adrenal hormonal functions, as it is composed only by adrenals. Increased levels of DHEA are common for women with PCOS. The DHEA-S is highest at a young age, so the age needs to be taken into consideration when doing the test. Patients who suffer from adrenal fatigue usually have lower levels of DHEA-S, while about 40-50% of the women suffering from the polycystic ovarian syndrome have increased levels of DHEA-S, that is related to the decreased egg quality.

5. Progesterone

The Progesterone is an important hormone of the hormonal cycle and plays a significant role during the second half of the cycle. It is secreted just after the ovulation has occurred. The Progesterone test is usually made on day 21, or in absence of regular menstruation on the 14th cycle day . If the levels are increased and higher than 16 nmol/L or 5 ng/ml it is an indicator that you have ovulated. If the levels of progesterone are low, you will feel anxious, and suffer from PMS and insomnia. Furthermore, it can cause heavy bleeding and difficulty with implantation.

6. Total Testosterone

The testosterone is produced mainly by the ovaries, although in certain quantities it can be produced adrenal glands as well. It is of vital importance for fertility and is also important for the muscle mass, boosting mood and libido, as well as increasing visual activity.

At a younger age women usually have increased levels of the testosterone, and it needs to be interpreted by taking women's age into consideration. Decreased levels of testosterone are common for patients that suffer from adrenal fatigue, and can make them feel tired and could feel a libido decrease. On the other side, increased levels of testosterone are typical for PCOS women who are also insulin influenced.The increased level of testosterone interrupts the menstrual cycle and the ovulation process.

The testosterone can also turn into estrogen through the process of aromatization, though the aromatization is not typical for PCOS patients and leads to inadequate follicle development.

The testosterone can also convert to a higher form of testosterone – DHT, that can lead to hair loss, hirsutism and skin problems as acne. There are various indicators for the testosterone as free and total testosterone, which reveal both the free floating and the produced testosterone. But, be careful! The testosterone solely can not be used for PCOS diagnosis as there can be normal levels of testosterone shown on the blood testing but there may be increased tissue levels of hormones that are not reflected in the blood.

7. Thyroid Stimulating Hormone (TSH)

The Thyroid Stimulating Hormone is also a pituitary hormone, which has a significant role in the thyroid hormone release. In case you have doubts that you might suffer from PCOS discuss with your doctor to also have a comprehensive laboratory test, and often the doctors will suggest to make a test only for the Thyroid Stimulating Hormone, but this is not enough to get a comprehensive overall picture about your thyroid health.

When it comes to values, usually anything higher than 3.0 mIU/l is an indicator for subclinical hypothyroidism. The American Thyroid Association advises an upper limit of 2.5 mIU/l for pregnancy.

8. Anti Mullerian Hormone

The anti mullerian hormone is an important hormone for women that want to conceive, as it counts the number of follicles presented in the ovaries, and it can help to anticipate the age of menopause.

As in some of the previous tests, also here the level of the Antimullerian hormone depends on the woman's age: younger women have increased levels of AMH, and the increased AMH equals to more follicles in the ovary. By the age of 33, the level of 2.1 -6.8 ng/ml of AMH is considered as normal. From 33 to 37 years old: 1.7 – 3.5 ng/ml, 38 to 40 years old: 1.1 – 3.0 ng/ml, while for over 41 years old, the level of AMH is around 0.5 – 2.5 ng/ml.

When it comes to fertility, for optimal fertility is considered AMH of 4.0 – 6.8 ng/ml, for satisfactory fertility is 2.2-4.0. Further decreasing as 0.3-2.2 ng/ml is sign for low fertility and 0.0-0.3 ng/ml for very low fertility. Decreased level of AMH means there are less follicles in the ovary and hence the lady most probably will need more time for conceiving, but still it is possible, and has been the case for plenty of women with low AMH to succeed to have a healthy pregnancy to term.

At any age, AMH level above 6.9 ng/ml is considered as an indicator for likely polycystic ovarian syndrome.

9. hs-CRP

High sensitive CRP or hs-CRP is not a hormone, but an indicator for the inflammation in the body. It is related to diverse health issues, such as weight gain, inflammation, autoimmunity, and of course, PCOS.

The hs-CRP test can show the extent of the inflammation at microvascular level. Patients that suffer from an autoimmune disease can have hs-CRP as high as 10, although a level of 2.0 is considered normal for healthy women. Even 3.0 level is already considered quite high.

10. Estradiol

It is recommended to take the estradiol test on the third day of the menstrual cycle, or alongside with the progesterone test on the 21st day of the cycle.

Higher levels of estradiol can decrease the FSH, hence leading to masked perimenopause and FSH levels. This happens in cases of functional cysts or low ovarian reserves. Interestingly, it also can be low in cases of menopause. Women with estradiol over 294 pmol/L Canadian units, or 80 pg/ml in US units, on the third day of the cycle, may have issues with the ovulation as the estrogen is being secreted on the cycle before, from the follicles that started developing early. This comes as a consequence of functional ovarian cyst or low egg quality, as the lower quality eggs are not in control to grow at the right rate, and develop too early.

You are not alone!

Being diagnosed with PCOS can be quite overwhelming at the beginning. Try to not isolate yourself and try to openly share with people you feel comfortable with. It is of vital importance to build a support group of positive people that can support you both emotionally and physically. Your team may include your partner, a friend, a colleague, dietician, doctors ect. You want people around you with whom you can openly communicate.

Fertility Clinic

After consulting your gynecologist, they might recommend a fertility clinic to assist you in further testing and possible fertility treatments. Do your research and choose the fertility clinic that you prefer. Most clinics have a website. Check their mission, the services they offer, the doctors etc. Also, most of them include their success rate, but do not rely too much on these statistics.

Support Group

A support group can be really helpful to get you through the treatments you will decide to do. Communicating with people who have been in the same situation, or have been through the same procedures, can really help ease the stress. Support groups are the place where you can express out loud your feelings and fears, and that will help you to dissociate yourself from your thoughts. Check if there is any in your area. If there is not, maybe you can discuss with a doctor about forming one!

Friends Support

Even though it might not be so easy to find others who are going through the same journey, that might not be the case. It is a sensitive topic, but try to reach and talk with your best friends. Understand their fertility journey! It might be something that could bring you closer together.

Naturopathic Doctor

Take into consideration to visit a naturopathic doctor. They can be very experienced in hormone balances, and might provide you support and advice when going through fertility treatment. A naturopathic doctor can collaborate with you to address any nutritional deficiencies, determine the underlying concern and promote an overall healthy environment for conceiving.

Counselor

When it comes to fertility management, it might be a struggle to accept the situation. It can provoke stress, feelings of doubts, mixed emotions and impatience. The worst thing you can do is to hold in your feelings. Reach out for an experienced counselor that can support you during this time. Also, some fertility clinics have them in their team, or can recommend you one.

Social Media

The power of social media also can not be underrated during this period. More and more people are looking to engage with other individuals that are in the same situation. It is a great way to connect with others and share your personal experience. Also, if you are worried about your privacy, by adjusting the privacy settings you can protect certain information, such as who can follow your journey, or who can interact with you.

Chapter 2: PCOS and Insulin

Probably you have realised by now that insulin resistance is not a good sign and is common for those women diagnosed with polycystic ovary syndrome. Still, the relation between PCOS and insulin resistance is not well defined. It is unclear whether the insulin resistance causes PCOS, or is the polycystic ovary syndrome that actually causes insulin resistance. Some studies have shown that PCOS is not caused by high insulin levels as the insulin only causes the release of androgens with PCOS women. Women that do not suffer from PCOS, they can be insulin resistant and can have completely normal androgens. Therefore the cause–effect relation is not defined, but still there is a lot that can be done. As more fatty tissue further irritates the insulin resistance, patients with the syndrome need to aim for a decreased BMI in order to promote optimal reproductive health.

But what is actually Insulin resistance?

Insulin resistance is a condition where the tissues and the cells become less sensitive to the insulin presented in the blood. As a consequence, the pancreas produces more insulin to achieve its main goal that is to prevent the blood sugar level to increase. Hence, there is a whole lot more insulin floating in the blood. Naturally, the insulin resistance happens with weight gain, or in case we are genetically predisposed and can lead to development of serious conditions such as diabetes, infertility, obesity and cardiovascular diseases. The typical signs for insulin resistance include weight loss resistance and abdominal fat gain. It influences 10% of young adults and around 44% of adults in mid-life.

Women with polycystic ovarian syndrome produce more testosterone when there is an increased presence of insulin. The extra testosterone decelerates the development of the follicles, leading to irregular menstrual periods, prolonged times for ovulation, and in severe cases it leads to infertility if the woman stops ovulating.

The insulin resistance can be measured by various methods. The hyperinsulinemic euglycemic clamp is considered gold standard for assessing the insulin resistance. It evaluates the level of glucose needed to compensate for the increased insulin in the blood. This is a difficult test to be performed, and hence is rarely performed in a clinic environment.

The second method is the HOMA-IR index which we mentioned previously, and that compares the levels of the fasting glucose and the fasting insulin. Simpler test that can be performed in a clinical setting is the test for HBA1C levels. This test can provide a good overview with regards to insulin resistance.

For PCOS, it is considered that there is a possible genetic defect inside the theca cells, the male hormone that produces cells, of the ovary. This leads the ovaries to produce higher quantities of male hormones when revealed to the insulin. It is common for patients with PCOS to have a family history of type 2 diabetes, or in some cases to have family relations of other women being diagnosed with PCOS.

As discussed previously, the insulin resistance is related to the high body mass index and the abdominal body fat that are connected to the fat that is accumulated near the organs and inside the abdominal activity. The abdominal fat deposits release free fatty acids more easily in comparison to the other parts of the body where fat is stored. The acids have an impact on the liver that produces LDL, the so-called bad cholesterol, releases glucose, and limits the removal of the insulin from the body.

The poor diet and unhealthy lifestyle can have an enormous impact on the insulin resistance in the body. Low fibre dishes, high fat and high carbohydrates have been constantly reported to induce insulin resistance.

Unhealthy high fructose drinks and snacks, as candy, soda and corn syrup products, provoke the liver to produce more triglycerides, that lead to metabolic syndrome related to serious health risks.

The polycystic ovarian syndrome is the most well-known insulin resistant condition that can seriously interrupt the female hormonal balance and has an impact on fertility. Fertility and insulin resistance are related by various links. Women that suffer from PCOS, their increased levels of insulin, affect the follicles in the ovaries producing androgens, which decelerates the development of the follicles and can even cause ovulation to completely cease.

Increased levels of insulin also cause fat cells to transform testosterone into estrogen, a process known as aromatization. Higher levels of estrogen increase the secretion of the LH – the luteinizing hormone, which leads to even more testosterone to be released by the ovaries. The estrogen also represses the FSH-follicle stimulating hormone which influences the eggs to not develop well.

Furthermore, insulin resistance decreases the SHBG – sex hormone binding globulin which binds together the hormones. When the level of the SHBG is low, there are a lot more androgens that are free, float in the bloodstream and produce androgenic effects.
It seems like a vicious cycle with no way to get out of it.

The high level of insulin is a typical cause of infertility and it contributes to miscarriage. Women suffering from PCOS and becoming pregnant are at increased risk of gestational diabetes, higher level incidence of Type II diabetes, preeclampsia, unfavourable lipid pattern, increased risk of cardiovascular disease and low bone density.

Insulin resistance and miscarriage

Women suffering from PCOS are at a high miscarriage risk when compared to women that do not suffer from the syndrome. Certain inflammatory factors have been found to be increased in women with PCOS, as C – reactive protein and homocysteine, which are also potential factors in implantation failure and miscarriage.

Insulin resistance also impacts the recurrent miscarriage. Research done with 74 women with recurrent pregnancy loss - rpl, showed that 27% of them had insulin resistance, compared to 9.5% of matched controls.

Insulin resistance and obesity

Women that suffer from PCOS and have gained weight have more infertility problems when compared to slim women that suffer from PCOS. This is the result of the increased BMI.
The increase of the BMI level to 27 and more is also influenced by the insulin resistance.
High levels of BMI are also related to higher blood and follicular leptin concentrations.
Leptin is a hormone that usually is exhibited at a higher circulating concentration in obese individuals that inhibits the apetite and helps to regulate the energy balance. Cells become resistant to leptin in cases of obesity, and the high levels of the leptin without the appropriate appetite control, certainly lead to more weight gain.
The leptin hormone also impacts the granulosa cells in the ovaries, and affects the function and quality of the follicles.

Furthermore, the lower serum adiponectin levels are also related with the increased BMI. The adiponectin is anti-inflammatory and impedes arterial plaques. It is a fat specific protein that has lower levels in patients suffering from cardiovascular diseases and type 2 diabetes. Obese women act in a similar way to the polycisic ovarian syndrome as it lowers the sex hormone binding globulin (SHBG).

Obesity also leads to chronic low-grade inflammation. Inflammation is related with various fertility conditions such as recurrent miscarriage and implantation failure. Research conducted on mouse models of obesity showed increased inflammatory markers CRP, interleukin-6 and TNF-alpha, all of which have been connected with infertility.

Insulin resistance and diabetes

Prediabetes is an epidemic condition. More than 1 out of 3 Americans, that would be around 84 million of American adults,have prediabetes. NIH estimates that is even higher for adults older than 65 – around 50%. And 90% of people do not know they have it!

If you suffer from PCOS and have high insulin resistance, it means increased risk of developing type 2 diabetes, stroke and heart disease. More than 50% of women that suffer from the polycystic ovarian syndrome develop type 2 diabetes by the age of 40. Gestational diabetes, diabetes when pregnant, also can lead to developing type 2 diabetes later in life, for both, the baby and the mother.

Diabetes, if not treated properly can lead to serious heart and kidney complications as well as to other serious issues.

If you have prediabetes, it is important that you pay attention to blood sugar numbers. Usually doctors do not communicate these numbers with their patients, unless they are really high. The normal level of the fasting glucose is 100. If you have it 100-125, it means that you have prediabetes. In case you are borderline, I would recommend that you make another test. You are not supposed to eat before the test.

Another test you can make is the test for Hemoglobin A1c, which is the 12 week average of the blood sugar. Fasting levels are not needed for this test. Normal level is below 5.7. From 5.7 to 6.4 it means you have prediabetes, while the diabetes start from 6.5 and higher.

If you have been diagnosed with low end of prediabetes, do not panic. It can be overwhelming, but you can prevent it, and even reverse it, by controlling the blood sugar through a suitable diet, lifestyle changes, exercises, and with medications if needed.

A major research, named the Diabetes Prevention Program, focused on researching if the oral diabetes drug Metformin (Glucophage) or diet and exercise could delay, or even prevent, the development of type 2 diabetes for people with Impaired Glucose Tolerance (IGT or prediabetes). 3.234 overweight and IGT diagnosed study participants have taken part in the research of the two very well-known factors that lead towards development of type 2 diabetes.

The first group participated in an intensive lifestyle training including: diet, exercising, and behavior modification. By consuming less fat and fewer calories and doing workout for a total of 150 minutes per week, the participants had to reach a goal of losing 7% of their body weight and also maintain it.

The second group took metformin, and another group was a placebo group.

The results showed that the diet modifications and the physical activity significantly decreased the chances up to 58% for the person with IGT to develop diabetes. The metformin also led to decreased risk for up to 31%.

The DPP solved these issues so quickly that, based on an external monitoring board advice, the program was terminated one year earlier. The experts published their findings on February 7, 2002, issued in the New England Journal of Medicine.

CHAPTER 3 NATUROPATHIC APPROACH FOR TREATING PCOS

So, if you already have been diagnosed with PCOS, and If have reached the stage where you have been trying to conceive, as often this is the phase PCOS is being diagnosed, you must felt that all your world has fallen apart, and is time to start introducing another term in your conversation with your partner, as IVF, surrogacy, and even adoption. But is it?

Doctors and researchers still can not define what causes PCOS. But it does not mean we need to wait for the cause to be diagnosed in order to treat it. What matters is that we learn to identify the symptoms and diagnose it, we learn how we deal with it, and we learn how to overcome it.

The treatment of the polycystic ovarian syndrome varies based on the individual characteristics of each patient, such as: the body type, the severity of the disease, metabolic characteristics, lab values and the level of inflammation. In some cases losing weight can help to improve the menstrual cycle. Also, the doctor may recommend taking a birth control pill, which can help to regulate the levels of hormones and establish hormone balance.

Of course, you should talk to your doctor before starting to take any medication or supplement. You may not be an adequate candidate to take a particular medication or your doctor may have recommended a specific regimen that will be more suitable for you. Feel free to ask your doctor about other alternatives, or why he or she recommends the suggested treatment, and if you have doubts regarding the treatment plan,discuss it with your doctor. The regime needs to be acceptable for both you and the doctor, and by openly communicating you should be able to find something that works for you. Various approaches can be helpful in different situations and at different periods of the woman's life. There are certain advantages and disadvantages of any kind of treatment.

For example, the Glucophage, also known as metformin, is usually used as oral medicine and can help you to establish a regular period on a structured basis. It is one of the most prescribed medicines, a part of the birth control pill, but it can provoke plenty of gastrointestinal side effects, that can be quite unpleasant. On the contrary, there are women that have severe symptoms, and the Metmorfin can be quite helpful. The inositol on the other hand, does not provoke side effects and for which benefits we will discuss more in the subsequent chapter, is used as a natural substitute for the patients that can not tolerate the Metformin.

The birth control pill is usually prescribed to calm the cysts in the ovaries, but it also covers the symptoms of PCOS which leads a lot of women to be undiagnosed. Moreover, another issue is that the pill leads to high clotting risk, that women with PCOS are already predisposed to. When they are young, they have irregular periods, so they are recommended to start taking birth control pills. They start to get regular periods, and so they never get to check their hormones. When they decide to have family, and get off the birth control pill, that is the time when they note the symptoms and are diagnosed with the polycystic ovarian syndrome. If they did not start taking the birth control pill most probably they would have noted the symptoms earlier.

I strongly believe that an integrative approach which combines the various types of treatments is the best option. I also believe that the patient needs to be aware of all treatments, be informed, and to make an informative decision of what she wants to use and what affects it will have on her body. That is why I invested so much time and effort in this book. The naturopathic approach takes a complete women's perspective treating individual symptoms, including: depression and anxiety, body gain issues, infertility and menstrual cycle regulation.Modalities involve lifestyle chances, nutritional supplements, acupuncture, diet and exercises, which will lead to sustainable solutions.

Acupuncture

Acupuncture has been indicated as one of the possible treatments that can treat the polycystic ovary syndrome and restore the natural ovulation in the female body. The treatment works to initiate the natural healing process by restoring the mental, physical and emotional disharmonies within the body. Research has shown 40 – 60% increase in success rate for IVF treatments.

It consists of acupuncture and electroacupuncture in the ovaries, that will lead to increase of the endorphins and endocrine, improve the immune functions of the body, tonifies the uterus, decreases inflammation, reduces stress and will improve significantly the blood circulation in the pelvic organs to prepare them for IVF or IUI cycles.

It can be used as an integrative method to the conventional approach for treating PCOS. Most probably, it will take a few months until the first signs of acupuncture sessions are felt and sessions can be extended to twice or more per week.

Moreover, acupuncture can be used to treat some common conditions such as: allergies, sinusitis, hypertensin, tinnitus, sore throats, gastroesophageal reflux, hyperacidity and peptic ulcer disease, depression and anxiety, dysmenorrhea, constipation, diarrhea, spastic colon, urinary incontinence, urinary tract infection, premenstrual syndrome, sensory disturbances other disorders.

It is a Chinese therapy that works for more than 2,500 years. It consists of insertion of thin needles at particular points of the body in order to balance the circulation of the energy, or the so-called "qi" through the various channels (meridians) in the body.

Although the thin needles tend to cause small discomfort when inserted, still the majority of the patients don't find the treatment painful, but have described that its rather an aching sensation that means it has been activated by the qi in the body. Furthermore, it is considered a safe process when trying to conceive. The diverse points work together to help activate the natural processes of your body, and will not interfere with any other processes or drugs you are getting when trying to conceive. Usually the needles will stay in for 25 to 35 minutes.

When it comes to the electro puncture, its effects have been investigated through neuropeptides, measurement of hormones and circulatory changes on both humans and animals who received this specific type of electro puncture. The electro puncture profoundly impacts the reproductive organs, through mechanisms in the endocrine systems, the neuroendocrine system, and the sympathetic nervous system. When the needles are inserted and stimulated into particular points, this results in a neurological reflex transferred to the organ that is related with that nerve pathway. As for example, the needles inserted into specific regions, as the lower back, abdomen or leg muscles below the knee provoke a response which significantly affects the ovary. In addition, the nervous system will transfer a signal to the brain, and the brain then emits a response which impacts the organ from the central mechanism. Furthermore, it has been found also that the electro puncture can decrease the high peripheral circulating ß-endorphins in women with the polycystic ovarian syndrome, and thereby improve insulin resistance.

How many treatments you will need, depends on the issues with which you are dealing and how serious it is. As the egg takes time to mature, sometimes it is needed for up to 3 months. But during an IVF treatment cycle, special dedication can be dedicated on specific acupuncture points to optimize the success rate.

When it comes to the cost of this treatment, it depends on the place where you live. It can range between 50-80 dollars. It might as well be covered by your health insurance. I know that Naturopathic insurance covers all acupuncture treatments.

So how does acupuncture actually help you?

1. In a situation of **hormonal imbalance,** a treatment focused on balancing yin and yang, will assure the ovulation and will decrease the androgen levels.

2. During **IVF treatments**, the acupuncture treatment timing Is different and arranged on the same day as the IVF treatment, or a day before it. Research has shown that the acupuncture contributes towards the egg quality and hence for improving the possibilities of successful pregnancies.

3. The acupuncture treatments concentrate on increasing the level of progesterone and assuring that the baby is receiving proper blood circulation, thus **preventing miscarriages.** Not a lot of studies has been done with regards to this aspect, but one study showed decrease in the early miscarriage symptoms, as vramping, back pain and bleeding.

4. Acupuncture treatments **tonifies the uterus** and also **decreases the inflammation** in the body, as through the various points in the body, the treatment reduces the release of the pro-inflammatory cytokines. The cytokines cause inflammation and pain in the body which affect conditions as the PCOS and endometriosis.

5. **Reduces stress and improves emotional well-being.**

According to the Chinese the Kidneys are responsible for our genetic makeup, that is known as our essence, and impacts the growth and development as well as the start of menstruation and menopause. The stress damages our adrenal glands and our kidneys. The situation of fright or stress is known as "scattering the qi." When the qi is scattered it cannot hold the embryo in the uterus. The acupuncture can tonify the kidneys in stressed situations so that the qi can flow smoothly in the body leading to a positive pregnancy outcome!

<u>What evidence exist for acupuncture inducing ovulation:</u>

Several researches were done on low frequency electroacupuncture and ovulation induction. In one study, was investigated the effect of a series of 14 electro acupuncture treatments on 24 anovulatory women who suffered from PCOS.

The regular ovulation is induced in 38% of them. LH/FSH ratios and the levels of the testosterone were significantly decreased three months after the last treatment.

Another research done on a group of lades given human menopausal gonadotropin, which is commonly used drug for treating infertility, acupuncture was compared to hCG injections in order to assess its impact on ovulation.

Traditionally hCG is used at fertility clinics during medicated processes in order to provoke ovulation. It was concluded that induced ovulation by a single acupuncture treatment can be as effective as the hCG injection and decrease the incidence of ovarian hyperstimulation syndrome. Some of the researches have also showed enhanced ovarian response when accupunture is used as addition to medicated cycles.

Another study included female rats with PCOS, induced by chronic exposure to the testosterone DHT. They were given physical exercise and low frequency electrocupuncture. The treatment lead to notably normalized cycles and higher quantity of healthy follicles.

Lifestyle changes

Hormones are chemical agents in the body, and each of them carries a specific task. In case of hormonal imbalance it means there is disintegration in the communication that can result with diverse unwanted symptoms. For establishing hormonal balance we can modify our lifestyle and establish healthy habits that will make us feel better and more energized.

So if until now, I focused on indicating a more general approach towards different aspects of PCOS, I would like to dedicate this chapter to sharing more practical tips. A lot of women find it hard to deal with the diagnosis and do not know how to proceed after that, or which should be the next step. Taking on a new set of habits can be simple with a small guide. Do not forget that it can be overwhelming to try to introduce all the new changes, and shock your organism. Start step by step and introduce new routines gradually. As to all other things, enjoy the transition process of your future-self.

Blood sugar control

Remember that it is necessary to keep a normal blood sugar level, as blood sugar constant changes can reduce other essential nutrients, impact the stress level in your body and your mood, and thus have consequences on your guts as well. Be mindful to not skip meals, include healthy fat and proteins in your dishes, consume healthy snacks and eat regularly throughout your day. Meal planning will be of great help with assisting you to keep the blood sugar under control.

Decrease caffeine

You do not have to completely eliminate the caffeine, just be more aware of how much you consume it and do not take it in excessive quantities as it can significantly increase the cortisol level and make you feel more stressed. Sometimes drinking coffee is more like a habitual ritual rather than a necessity. You can also try to substitute coffee with herbal teas that can have beneficial effects for your body.

The Dandy Blend which contains dandelion, rye, chicory, barley and beet roots, tastes like coffee but it is caffeine and gluten-free and can also substitute the coffee and might be a good choice especially for those that are addicted to the taste of coffee.

Other options can involve the turmeric latte, decaf coffee and adaptogen latte.

Pay attention to your daily cups of coffee and make a research of which option might suit you best.

Eat healthy fat

Yes, fat can be not healthy in certain cases, but you need to differentiate healthy to unhealthy fat. The avocado oil, olive oil, olives, coconut, nuts, seeds, coconut oil, fatty fish as salmon are great sources of healthy fats which are needed for hormone system function and for stress level regulation.

Detoxification

Detoxication or detoxification is the elimination of the toxic substances from the body, and it happens through the liver function. Although some scientists have described the diet detox as non-functional due to the lack of scientific research, still in alternative medicine, it is widely promoted. Patients are encouraged to reduce the consumption of environmental toxics, to eat organic when possible, drink more water, and to try to consume more cruciferous veggies as kale, broccoli and cauliflower.

Quality sleep

Sleep is of great importance for physical and mental well-being and regulates the quantity of cortisol production.

Try to establish a solid routine that will prepare your body for bedtime, such as trying to prepare for bed at the same time each day, limit the screen time, have dinner a few hours before going to bed, dim the light etc. This will help you to improve the quality of sleep and you will wake up more energized the next day.

Try to eliminate the use of electronics, including your cell phone for at least one hour before you go to bed. The blue light from the electronic gadget can affect the biorhythm, and the messages and constant reading of news can be quite distracting. Calming herbal teas as lemon balm, lavender, chamomile can help you to relax before going to bed.

Having a bath or taking a shower before going to bed also can be quite effective for improving your sleep. Hot water alongside with a few drops of essential oils can help you to melt away the stress from the day and put your body in a relaxing mood before you go to bed.

The use of Epsom salt can be beneficial because it contains magnesium that will have an impact on your muscles and will help to relax them.

While it might be difficult and you will need some time to establish and adapt to a night routine, try to keep it as regular as possible, even during the weekends. Each body functions in its own way, and rest time will be different for each person, but ideally you would try to have 7-8 hours of night sleep.

Avoid stress

The stress started to have a huge impact on our lives as it is normal to experience daily stressful situations.It is something that one of us experiences, and in small amounts it keeps us going and gives us energy and motivation. One the other hand, higher amounts of stress can significantly impact our health.Often stress can trigger hormone imbalances, as the body will do whatever is necessary to cope with a threat. It is of particular importance to dedicate time to transitioning our nervous system into parasympathetic mode. This mode is present when we are relaxed and feel safe, and promotes digestive function, sleep, healing and proper neurotransmitter balance.

Try to avoid stress as much as possible and also, try to apply various coping strategies such as: practice mindfulness, meditation, journaling etc. that will help you in times of stress and anxiety.

Useful tips to reduce stress:

- Family relations and friendships are extremely important in these situations. Reaching out to an old friend, and having a nice cup of coffee together, or chatting via video calls will instantly improve your mood. This kind of human relation will help a lot in the process of stress relief.

- If you feel the need to ask for professional help, as a trusted counselor or a psychologist, that will make a world of difference for stress alleviation.

- Being informed is essential , but in certain periods can be incredibly overwhelming if you are constantly checking your phone and scrolling through the social networks, and being continually focused on bad news and arguments. Limit the time you spend on the social networks, and check them just once or twice per day. Mute notifications as well as they can make you feel particularly stressed when interrupted during your daily tasks, and might tempt you to check the phone.

- Try to dedicate a few minutes per day to journaling. Writing down your thoughts each day can significantly improve your mental health and how you deal with stress. I advise you to use a handwritten journal instead of online, as the brain-emotional connection is stronger. You will become more self conscious as you start exploring your ideas. Filling the blank pages will clear your mind from the stressed thoughts that make you feel anxious.

- Take time for yourself: relax by watching a good movie, read a book, spend some time relaxing in nature, workout or dedicate some time on your hobby. Certain hobbies as adult coloring and drawing, needlework and knitting can significantly contribute to relaxing yourself.

Practice mindfulness

Daily stress and daily worries can often make you feel anxious. Mindfulness can help us to not constantly hold on to thoughts that keep on reappearing and can be the key for helping us to release anxiety. Meditation is about allowing the thought to drift away.

I know it is not easy to start with and it takes time and practice. But if you can dedicate just 10 to 20 minutes daily, you will get to see the difference soon and can make a big difference in how you feel.

I know that sometimes it can be difficult to find the time, but just close the door and simply sit and try to relax. Add some essential oils to the diffuser, such as geranium, orange, and lavender. Enjoy the scent of the oil and help your body and mind to forget about all the daily stress. Pay attention to your breathing, as during the workouts also throughout the day. We have the habit to often breathe shallowly during the day. It is important to improve your breathing as the deep breathing can reduce tension and fight stress. When you take deep breaths, your body communicates to your mind and it gives signals to relax and calm down.

 If you are just starting with meditation I can recommend some applications that can be of great help:

- Online Restorative Yoga Classes;
- Headspace App that offers guided meditation and mindfulness;
- Calm App;
- Circle and Bloom that offers as well some free options and is specific to women's health, fertility and pregnancy.

Workout

Workout can be a great way to manage the anxious energy and reduce stress, it can also improve fertility for women who have PCOS mostly through reducing the waist circumference and weight loss. Moderate intensity workout programs as Pilates, yoga ect. can have significant impact on reducing the high level of cortisol The poor micro vascular uterine functions is also common typical for women with PCOS, and can lead to implantation failure. Exercise training may improve the micro vascular function by enhancing nitric oxide vasodilation.

A research conducted with 40 obese women with anovulatory PCOS showed that structured exercise lead to improved menstrual regularity, fertilty and insulin sensitivity. The structured exercise program consisted of 30 minutes stationary bicycle sessions, three times per week.

So, try to introduce exercise to your daily routine. 30 minutes per day is more than enough. Although it might seem easy, I know you might be struggling to find time for it or how to start. I recommend you to begin by gradually introducing it in your daily habit, and to stick to one golden rule : NEVER MAKE EXCEPTIONS FOR MORE THAN ONE TIME! So if you decided to workout 3 times per week at the beginning, you can not skip the workouts for two subsequent times.

Yoga aims to lengthen and extend our muscles, and also regulates our breathing, therefore it can significantly contribute towards tension decrease in our body and calm the anxious thoughts. Another app for yoga that you can try is Yoga Studio by Gaia.

Change your eating habits

Your diet and eating habits make a huge difference in various ways. If you are overweight, just by reducing your body weight for 5-10% can have a great impact in your battle against PCOS. It will help you to establish regular menstrual cycles and decrease the symptoms as acne and facial hair.

When it comes to PCOS, special attention should be given to insulin resistance which causes the ovaries to produce testosterone. Whenever we eat, the level of the blood sugar increases, and the insulin is released in order to deal with the blood sugar. But, as explained previously, in case of polycystic ovarian syndrome there is an increased amount of released insulin, so there is way more insulin in the body. It is important to pay attention to the type of food you take and how often you eat.

Everything matters: the quantity, type of food, quality of the products, inflammatory property and calorie density. By choosing foods that secrete less insulin, you will see improvements in the syndrome symptoms. Try to keep your blood sugar under control by eating often and in small portions. Your meals and snacks need to include proteins and good fats that can be found at the hummus dip, seeds and seeds butter, as well as with nuts and nuts butter.

Plan 6-7 servings per day of meals full with vegetables out of which two are leafy greens, and include daily serving of lentils or black beans. Including one or two tbsp. of cinnamon in your breakfast meal each day and it will help to increase the insulin sensitivity.

Limit the fruit consumption and replace it with low glycemic index fruit as the berries.

Be careful with the portion size which can influence the insulin resistance and the glucose load. Reduce at minimum the intakes of milk and dairy products, in case you prefer a non-vegan diet, carbohydrates as sugar and any type of flour, including also the products made with them: bread, pasta, muffin, biscuits etc.

Chapter 4: DIET and PCOS

Modern medicine does not often think that the diet can make much of a difference, but slowly everyone is changing their mind. In 2013, one of the American biggest groups of reproductive specialists, shared a committee opinion stating that there is not a lot of evidence with regards to how vitamin enriched diet, dietary variations, herbal medicines, or antioxidants can improve fertility. After four years, they changed their mind, stating that emerging epidemiologic data showed that the diet can impact reproductive health.

Moreover, translational work with animal models and human specimens lends biologic plausibility to the epidemiologic data, specifically in the context of female reproductive diseases related with PCOS, obesity and inflammation.

When such a conservative group changed their opinion after just 4 years, it seems that we are starting a new era when modern medicine will start paying more attention to the diet and the eating habits.

Food to avoid

Avoiding certain types of food can significantly contribute to reverse your PCOS. Plenty of standard comfort food contains ingredients that provoke havoc in PCOS symptoms. I am not insinuating to eliminate them all at once, as I understand it can be quite overwhelming. I would rather see it as an ongoing process, a transformation that will take time but will lead to a more sustainable solution. Start by slowly replacing them to healthier alternatives, and you will see the lasting impact on your health and wellbeing.

Avoid Dairy

I know, I know….cheese is amazing! I adore it too and was one of the products that made it the most difficult for me to switch to vegan diet.

But vegan cheese is great as well! And it does not come together with the dairy protein that highly increases the insulin. Actually, for a while, I have been quite passionate about making a guide of how to make your own plant based milk and cheese from scratch at home. It is really simple and you can experiment a lot with it in the kitchen!

Beside the dairy proteins, USA dairy often includes growth hormones, concentrated quantities of environmental toxins, like glyphosate, and pesticides have also been found. Furthermore, many people have dairy allergies or are lactose intolerant and are not even aware of it. These products lead to low-grade inflammation in the body, aggravating autoimmune conditions like rheumatoid arthritis.

There are also the low-fat dairy products, for which people do not think they are related with insulin resistance. A study conducted in Iran, monitored 1205 participants for more than 2 years, showed that the BCAA – the Branched Chain Amino Acids, which are present in very high quantities in a varios dairy products, are huge triggers and can cause insulin resistance.

The Branched Chain Amino Acids can be often found in products as whey powder, that is used for protein drinks and smoothies, and in the low-fat dairy products, as low-fat cheese, low-fat or fat-free yogurt and kefir, low-fat milk as well as in the skim milk. When these products are consumed during a sedentary period, instead of after an intense workout, they add on fat storage rather than muscle tissue.

Avoid Sugar

Sugar tastes good, but for sure does not have a lot of redeeming qualities. It causes an immediate blood sugar spike, followed by a solid crash. The insulin increases as well, and leads to cascade effect, as when the insulin level increases, the ovaries start releasing testosterone. When the insulin levels remain high for a longer period of time, t fat burning slows down exponentially. Moreover, sugar also disrupts the bacterial balance inside our intestines, changing the types of microorganism species that are present inside.

Try to switch the sugar with healthy fats, nutrient-dense protein and non-starchy vegetables. If you are at a gathering, and someone offers to try the dessert they prepared, just try it and you will get to indulge without taking too much sugar.

Avoid wheat and flour products

The modern Western diet involves too much grains and carbohydrates. Do you remember the food pyramid that many of us studied at school? It showed that 5-7 servings of breads, cereals and grains was ok for good health.

Though, a different type of food pyramid is needed. One that focuses on leafy and non-starchy vegetables.

The majority of the flour products have a high glycemic index, which means that they get rapidly converted into sugar. Grains such as: rye, spelt, wheat and barley are the ones that contain gluten, and contain also inflammatory substances such as gliadin. This substance is really problematic for people that suffer from the Celiac disease, but it can be irritating to the non-Celiacs as well. Gluten can lead to leaky gut as well as immune reactions. In case you have doubts that you might be sensitive to gluten, try eliminating it for a month and see how you feel. If you feel better overall, try to avoid it in the future! If that is not the case, then most likely you are not too sensitive to it. So if you do not suffer from the Celiac disease, occasionally you can use wheat or grain products. Still, North American wheat products tend to be highly processed, while the European wheat products tend to be more tolerant as those countries use a different variety known as soft wheat which contains less gluten. Softer gluten means it is easier to break down.

One of the common questions I come across is: "Do carbohydrates themselves cause inflammation?" Yes, and no. When the level of blood sugar increases, the immune system replies by producing an elevated number of reactive oxygen species. These damaging chemicals are released as the mitochondria, the cell's internal powerhouses, work to store and use the sugar through particular metabolic pathways.

How much inflammation is produced after a carbohydrate-heavy meal depends on two factors: how high blood sugar levels get and how long the blood sugar remains high after consuming food. Moreover, anything that notably increases the insulin levels will also contribute to the higher insulin resistance. If a meal is high in refined carbohydrates, lower in fibre and healthy fats, and has a high insulin or glycemic index, it will cause a relatively large spike in blood sugar after the meal. The body then declines into a pro-inflammatory state as the mitochondria fight to manage this excessive carbohydrate-derived energy.

It is important to know that the fructose, which has a low glycemic index, through completely different mechanisms in the liver generates 100 times more reactive oxygen species than the glucose. Therefore, consuming fruits in large quantities or sweetened foods are equally problematic for inflammation.

You do not have to give up on delicious food products. It's just a matter of swapping it for healthier options, such as using spiralized zucchini or spaghetti squash instead of grain-based pasta noodles.

You can still enjoy delicious meals, without blood sugar spikes.

Avoid Diet Sodas and Artificial Sweeteners

The diet industry is trying to make us believe that zero-calorie diet sodas are a better option instead of a normal soda, and are absolutely okay to consume. After all, it says zero calories, so we can not gain any weight. Totally wrong! The artificial sweeteners are part of the diet of soft drinks, which do far more harm than most people think. By damaging the blood vessels, these sweet chemicals can cause obesity and metabolic disorders. Research has shown that by affecting the brain's prefrontal cortex, they reduce the impulse control, which literally makes it more difficult for people to refuse sweets. So, not that they are not helping in weight loss, but they also make it harder for the people to avoid eating foods high in calories, such as cakes, cookies and ice cream.

Try to replace these drinks with healthier options, as herbal tea, green tea and homemade vegetable juices .

Avoid Packaged Foods

Once back from the supermarket check the ingredients list of the pre-packaged items that you bought. How many of them can you recognize or pronounce? They contain artificial flavours, processed flour, sugars and preservatives, as well as ingredients that are high in calorie, but do nothing to nourish your body. So they will just increase the blood sugar levels and you will feel energised at the very same moment, but that energy will significantly drop after a while. By reducing the consumption of these products plenty of different health problems will be sustained. Switch these for whole foods items, as found in nature! Cook from scratch, with natural ingredients, and do not buy anything that your great grandmother would not have recognized as food. You will shortly notice immediate improvement.

I know sometimes it can be difficult to dedicate time to cooking due to busy daily schedules and stressed life, but cooking in bulk and freezing meals, can be of great help! For me it worked to dedicate part of the weekend on planning the meals for the next week, so I do not have to worry for the meals, or eat outside if too tired to cook.

What about alcohol?

Having a cocktail or glass of wine is part of socializing. But there are some drinks that are preferably chosen over other ones.Sugar in cocktails comes from the mixer , not from real alcohol. Also the distilled alcohol and the wine start out being high in carbs or sugar, found in grain and grapes, even though the carbohydrates and the sugar, with the process of fermentation, are converted to alcohol. Distilled alcohol like vodka, gin or rum or gin have about 100 calories for 1.5 oz. White wine or dry red has about 125 calories per 5ox glass, and about 4 grams of carbs. Studies that included people with type 1 or type 2 diabetes and who drank moderate amounts of alcohol alongside food, showed no alcohol effects on insulin levels or on blood sugar.

Still, sweet wines and beer can contain more carbs, so try to avoid them, and opt dry white and red wine, or unsweetened alcoholic drinks as vodka with soda and fresh limon. Try to take a glass of water between the alcoholic drinks as well.

So although alcohol can make part of a PCOS friendly diet, still It can be different for every person. I advise you to pay attention on how it impacts your body, like: mood changes, energy levels and sleep quality.

Plant based diet for PCOS

There are various diets that can help PCOS. There is not a single one that guarantees you the results you need. Diverse diets work for different people that are diagnosed with PCOS. It can be the Meditteranean diet, the Ketogenic diet, low glycemic index diet, or the one I included in this research, and is often used in some of the most developed clinics dedicated to PCOS, the food insulin demand diet. Products that just increase insulin will obviously worsen things. We don't want to further increase the insulin level of what is now. Medicine is developing a lot and there have been profound changes noticed in medicine's approach towards diet and nutrition.

Do not do diets! Focus on healthy eating and nutritional meals! Embrace the whole grain source of carbohydrates. Whole food, strawberry, lemon are the best.

Do not skip meals! Skipping breakfast, or any other meal will not help you at all. If you skip a meal, your body will struggle to process the sugar. In order to constantly keep the blood sugar under control,plan your meals well in advance, including much needed snacks. If you are out of home for a longer time, take a prepared snack with you. Assure that your stomach is not completely empty, nor completely full as it might be a problem to digest the food. Might be tricky to establish this habit at the beginning, but trust me,in the long term it gets really easy, and it becomes a habit. Balancing will keep the sugar under control and help you fight against insulin resistance.

Fill the fridge and the pantry with fresh fruit and vegetables. Do not substitute the fruit with fruit juice! Whole fruits contain fibers. Consume the good types of fats, and slowly introduce to your diet, all the spices we have discussed previously.

The easiest way to do this is to stop buying the products you are supposed to avoid. If you live with your family or your partner, explain your struggle to them, why and what you need to do and see how they can be of a support to you.

Do not expect them to understand and change their own habits as of tomorrow, just because you decided to eat healthy.

So, can a plant-based diet help for PCOS?

When we say plant-based, some of you might think that a bowl of white pasta with vegetables might be ok as they come from plants. But what is important to pay attention to is that you need a whole foods plant based diet! Diet that eliminates animal products and includes unrefined and wholesome plant sources such as fruits, vegetables, beans, whole grains, seeds, nuts and legumes. It focuses on minimally processed foods and avoids refined foods like white flour, added sugar and refined oils. Still, keep in mind there is no one single definition of a plant based diet.

Plant based diets may offer additional benefits as they are full of nutrients including fibers, folate, phosphorus, Vit B6 and Vit C, potassium, magnesium and beta-carotene. Of course, this refers to eating a balanced plant based diet.

It has been found that plant based diets can improve many health conditions related to polycystic ovarian syndrome, including: inflammation, risk of heart disease, insulin resistance, type 2 diabetes, cholesterol, weight gain and promote healthier gut microbiome. (Dr. Felice Gersh is doing some great research if you want to check).

A review study from the Diabetes & Metabolic Syndrome: Clinical Research & Reviews, in 2017, published that *"A favorable dietary plan for women with PCOS should contain low amounts of saturated fatty acids with average amounts of saturated fatty acids with one double bond and omega-3. Additionally, sufficient intake of fiber-rich diet from whole grains, legumes, vegetables and fruits with an emphasis on carbohydrate sources with low glycemic index is highly recommended."* Seems like a plant based diet, right?

Research conducted with more than 300 000 people, out of which 24

000 had diabetes, showed that plant-based foods, as whole grains, legumes, nuts, vegetable and fruit can lead to 30% decrease in the risk of type 2 diabetes. Take into consideration that the focus of the research was only to the relation, not to the cause and effect, and it did not show explicitly why a plant-based diet leads to decreased type 2 diabetes risk. Probably the reason is that people who have a plant-based diet may maintain a healthier weight and the beneficial compounds, like antioxidants and beneficial plant oils, help reduce inflammation and promote insulin sensitivity. Also, with the plant-based diet you directly avoid animal products, and hence also the sodium and saturated fats. Furthermore, plant based dishes can have a favorable effect on the gut microbiome, which can lead to decreased insulin resistance.

Still, although the plant-based diets are wholesome and abundant in vegetables, fruits and legumes, there are some nutrients of concern, as calcium, iron, protein, choline, vitamine B12, that you should be aware of before embarking on a plant-based lifestyle. You can still obtain these nutrients with planning and maybe supplementation. So be sure to get informed before you start or if possible, you as well can ask for the help of a nutritionist at the beginning so you can be sure that you are having balanced dishes.

Natural Supplements for PCOS

There is a variety of natural supplements that can manage the signs of polycystic ovary syndrome. As there is insulin resistance, there is a lot of mineral deficiency in PCOS. The natural supplements can decrease the level of testosterone and contribute towards the regulation of the menstrual cycles as well as of the ovulation in women with PCOS.

Inositol

The inositol is a supplement similar to vitamin B, and can help to treat diverse symptoms of PCOS. It can be found in two forms: myo-inositol and d-chiro-inositol (DCI).

- A research conducted with 50 PCOS patients that do not have ovulation, showed that the inositol can help to reduce the insulin resistance, and also to improve the function of the ovaries.
- The combined therapy of D-Chiro inositol and Myo has proved effective in decreasing the level of testosterone, in order to establish a regular menstruation cycle. Myo-inositol combination may as well help to decrease the level of incompatible eggs in the patients that fight with infertility, and hence to fight the infertility and boost ovulation.
- Triglycerides are a type of fats that are the main components of body fat in the umans, and are also stored into our blood. When the body is not able to use the sugar and convert it into energy, as in case of insulin resistance, it will convert it into triglycerides and their presence in the blood will increase. High levels of triglycerides are dangerous and present increased risk for heart strokes and artery diseases. Inositol helps to reduce the levels of triglyceride. D-chiro inositol has

been proven to increase insulin sensitivity, and hence to decrease the level of triglycerides in the blood.

- The inositol can play an important role also in fighting gestational diabetes that can be developed by patients who already suffer from PCOS, and derives as a consequence of the ability of the inositol to improve the insulin sensitivity, and hence prevent the risk of developing gestational diabetes.

Cinnamon

The benefits of cinnamon have been the core of numerous studies. Cinnamon is a supplement rich with polyphenolics and has been used in the Chinese medicine for decreasing the fasting blood glucose and also in insulin sensitivity improvement. You can sprinkle it on some of your dishes and easily incorporate it in your diet.

Chromium

Chromium is a mineral, needed in small amounts, and the level of it can decrease with the age. Chromium can be found in liver, broccoli, potatoes, red wine, brewers' yeast and green beans. It can be beneficial for losing weight or building muscle. Recently, further systematic researches have been conducted and concluded that the chromium can contribute in treating the insulin issues, decreasing the BMI, and can put the blood sugar under control. Still, be careful and do not take it without previous consultation with a nutritionist or doctor, as often is not recommended to be taken during pregnancy or in case of breastfeeding.

Magnesium

Magnesium is a mineral and it can be found in different food products, as spinach, spices, oats, nuts, cocoa and many others. Also it can be found as a dietary supplement in the pharmacies. Magnesium can help treat insulin resistance, blood sugar control and glucose metabolic disorders.

Turmeric

The turmeric is a spice that can be found in many Asian cuisines, especially in the cuisines of Malaysia, Iran, Polynesia, Thailand, India and China. It is known due to its anti-inflammatory and antioxidant effects that can have an impact on insulin regulation and also can help in the fight against a variety of diseases including the polycystic ovary syndrome.

Omega-3

The omega-3 are fatty acids that can be taken as supplement, or found in the diverse food products, as fish, walnuts, flaxseed and chia seeds. The omega-3 can be helpful in numerous ways in fighting the symptoms of PCOS: it can decrease the triglycerides, fight against insulin resistance, fight against the anxiety, treat hair loss and acne problems.

Omega-3 fatty acids are natural ligands of PPAR-Gamma receptors which have a significant role in controlling lipid metabolism. The PPAR-Gamma receptors also obstruct the inflammatory gene expression.

Research was conducted in 2018 including 60 women diagnosed with polycystic ovarian syndrome. They were given omega-3 fatty acid, 2x1000mg/day fish oil or placebo for 3 months. The final evaluation was that fish oil led to better insulin regulations, decreased inflammatory markers –HS-CRP, improved hirsutism, and had beneficial effects on mental health as well.

N-acetylcysteine (NAC)

N-acetylcysteine is a medication that can be used as dietary supplement as well as it has effects on boosting ovulation of women that suffer from PCOS and have infertile problems, and can also positively affect the endometrial thickness.

Zinc

Zinc is a trace element that can be found in meat, legumes, seeds and fish. It can be beneficial for treating unwanted hair growth, as well as hair loss, to treat skin issues, as acne are one of the symptoms of PCOS, improve the blood sugar control, improve the ovulation, as well as to support the work of the thyroid.

Herbal teas for treating PCOS

In various ways the herbal teas can improve our overall physical and mental health, and they can be also helpful in fighting the polycystic ovary symptoms in a natural way. And they can help with more than just one PCOS symptom! The most useful herbs are those with blood sugar stabilising properties, anti-inflammatory and cleansing powers, as well as having a high antioxidant structure to protect cells from being damaged. So, maybe it is time to consider switching your afternoon coffee ritual to a nice herbal tea.

White peony tea

The white peony tea, also known as Bai Muda, is slightly oxidized tea that affects the conversion of testosterone into estrogen thanks to its constituent named paeoniflorin. As a consequence, by lowering the testosterone, the ovulation is improved.

Cinnamon tea

As mentioned, cinnamon helps treat insulin levels and blood sugar levels. Numerous studies have confirmed the benefits of the cinnamon in fighting PCOS symptoms and taking it in the form of a tea can facilitate its incorporation in our eating habits. It can be made with cinnamon powder or just simply boiling cinnamon sticks. Besides treating the polycystic ovarian syndrome symptoms, it can also help reduce the risk of heart diseases, treat yeast infections, preserve brain functions etc.

Red reishi tea

The reishi mushroom also known as lingzhi mushroom, grows in wet and hot places in Asia, and in the eastern medicine is used for boosting the immune system, fighting depression, fighting cancer. It also has significant impact on decreasing the androgens, as the testosterone, while the red reishi can influence the transformation of the testosterone to dihydrotestosterone (DHT), which consequently influences the hair loss and the skin issues, as the acne.

Dandelion root tea

The dandelion root tea is a great herbal tea for treating the polycystic ovarian syndrome as it helps to detoxify the liver, which has a significant role in establishing hormonal balance.

Nettle tea

Nettle, also known as urtica dioica, significantly affects blood sugar control and decreases testosterone. It was shown in a study conducted with 40 women who experienced increased levels of androgen. As a consequence, it also helped with treating the symptoms related with increased testosterone, as hirsutism, acne and hair loss.

Spearmint tea

Spearmint tea is also great herbal tea for treating PCOS, as researches showed that the spearmint tea can help to increase follicle stimulating hormone, luteinizing hormone (LH) and estradiol. The ovulation process also improves, s it impacts the follicular development in the ovaries.

Chamomile

The chamomile is one of most popular members of the *Asteraceae* family, used for over 5 000 years. It is noted as calming botanical medicine, but has plenty of other benefits as well, as the anti-inflammatory effect.

A study has been conducted with 80 women suffering from PCOS. In a period of 3 months they were given 370 mg of chamomile capsules, 3 times per day. Another control group received placebo. After the 3 months period, an improvement has been noticed of the triglycerides and lipids as the LDL, in the group that took the herb. The ratio between the FSH and the LH also ameliorated and has been noted as a decrease of the level of testosterone.As an addition, the chamomile can also affect the brain's master hormonal regulation effects.

Chapter 5: Recipes

This Chapter, Chapter 7, I see it as a little gem of this book. It includes 40 plant-based, highly nutritious recipes that you can use as inspirations, and incorporate into your healthy eating and healthy living lifestyle. Healthy lifestyle is what we aim for. That is why it's necessary to find time for preparing and enjoying the meals, and not live through the experience as "something you are forced to do!"

Breakfast:

Often breakfast food contains carbs that can spike your insulin. Still, by slightly changing the recipes, you can still have your morning cake or enjoy the comfort of a delicious oatmeal without worrying about the blood sugar spike.

1. Vegan Nutella Overnight Oats

Servings: 1

Preparation time: 5 minutes

Refrigeration time: 6-8 hours

INGREDIENTS

- 45g old-fashioned gluten-free rolled oats
- 15ml homemade "Nutella" or hazelnut butter
- 125 ml plant-based milk
- 7 g cocoa or cacao powder
- 7 g ground flaxseed

Optional:

- Chopped dairy-free dark chocolate
- Strawberries
- Sea salt
- Hemp seeds

Instructions:
01. Mix all the ingredients in an air-tight jar the night before. Leave them overnight in the fridge
02. The next morning just take it out of the fridge, add the desired toppings and enjoy your meal!

Tip: In an air-tight container, can stay up to 2 days in the fridge. This meal can stay up to 2 days in the fridge if placed in an air-tight container.

2. Coconut and tropical mango overnight oats

Servings: 1

Preparation time: 5 minutes

Refrigeration time: 6-7 hours

Ingredients:
- 7g chia seeds
- 125 ml plant based milk
- 65g old fashioned gluten-free oats
- 165g fresh diced mango
- 15 mL almond butter
- ½ tsp pure vanilla extract

Optional:
Fresh fruit: strawberries, mango, kiwi, blueberries

Coconut flakes

Almond butter

Instructions:
01. Put all the ingredients in an air-tight jar the night before. Leave them overnight in the fridge
02. The next morning just take it out of the fridge, add the desired toppings and enjoy!

Tip: In an air-tight container can stay up to 2 days in the fridge.

3. Sweet potatoes wraps

Servings: 4

Preparation time: 10 minutes

Cooking: 15 minutes

Ingredients:

For the sweet potatoes:

- 2 sweet potatoes
- 40g frozen peas
- 5ml coconut oil
- 1/2 tsp ground coriander
- 1/2 tsp ground cumin
- 1/2 tsp turmeric powder
- Salt and pepper

For the tofu scramble:

- 225 g medium or firm tofu
- 1 diced onion
- 5 ml coconut oil
- 1 tsp garlic powder
- 1 tsp nutritional yeast
- 1 tsp turmeric
- Salt and pepper to taste

For the wrap:
- Sliced red bell pepper

- Sliced avocado
- Whole wheat wraps

1. Cut the sweet potatoes into 1inch cubes.
2. Steam the potatoes in a pot for 10-15 minutes, over high heat. Check with a fork if they are ready.
3. Heat the coconut oil the onions. Fry it quickly until it gets soft.
4. Squeeze the water from the tofu, break it with hands and add it to the onions.
5. Add the nutritional yeast, turmeric, garlic powder, the salt, and pepper to taste.
6. Proceed to cook for another 3 minutes until everything is mixed well.
7. Once ready, remove from the heat.
8. Now is time to get back to the potatoes. Melt the coconut oil in a pan and add the drained sweet potatoes.
9. Mash the potatoes with a fork and add the peas and the spices.
10. Mix well all ingredients and remove from the heat.
11. Put together the wraps: add the tofu scramble, potato filing, as well as the sliced avocado and red peppers. Enjoy!

The sweet potatoes and scrambled tofu wraps can be stored in the fridge for 3 days. You can enjoy it while hot or let everything cool off.

Tip: the sweet potatoes can be replaced with regular potatoes.
If you are using organic products, you can as well keep the skin of the regular potatoes for extra fibres!

4. Green Matcha Smoothie

Servings: 4

Preparation time: 5 minutes

Ingredients:

- 380 mL light coconut milk
- 250 ml plant-based milk
- 7g matcha powder
- 2 frozen bananas
- 250g fresh or frozen pineapple
- 40g leafy greens: spinach or kale
- 30g hemp seeds
- 4 dates

<u>Optional:</u>

Coconut flakes;

Blueberries;

Pineapple;

Strawberries;

Orange.

DIRECTIONS

Put all ingredients in a high-speed blender. Blend until they are well combined.

Add the toppings you prefer and enjoy!

5. Beginner's Green Smoothie

If you never tried, most probably just the thought of Green Smoothie reminds you of the taste of green leafy vegetables. I do not judge you! I was thinking the same! For those who never tried it, the green smoothie is gross by default. That is why I included this green smoothie for beginners in this book. Give it a try!

Servings: 1

Preparation time: 5 minutes

INGREDIENTS

- 2 peeled and frozen bananas
- 30g fresh spinach
- 30g peanut butter
- 375mL plant milk (I used almond milk made at home)

Optional:

Peanuts

Almonds

Chia

DIRECTIONS

Put all ingredients in a high-speed blender. Blend until they are well combined.

Add the toppings you prefer and enjoy!

6. Immune – Booster Smoothie

Yield: 2 servings

Total Time: 5 min

INGREDIENTS

- 2 frozen bananas
- peeled orange
- 50 g frozen raspberries
- 30 g raw spinach
- ¼ raw peeled beetroot
- 1-inch chunk fresh ginger
- 15 mL nut butter (I used peanut butter)
- 250 mL plant-based milk
- 60 mL plant-based yogurt (I used coconut)

<u>Optional toppings</u>

Granola

Nuts

Chia seeds

Toasted coconut flakes

Fresh berries

DIRECTIONS

Put all ingredients in a high-speed blender and pulse until well combined.

Once ready, put it into bowls, add the toppings you desire and enjoy!

7. Chia Pudding

Servings: 2

Prep Time: 5 min

Total Time: 1-2 hrs (refrigeration time for chia seeds to gel)

INGREDIENTS: THE PUDDING

- 45g chia seeds
- 5 chopped roughly dates
- 250mL plant-based milk
- 8g cocoa powder
- 1 tsp pure vanilla extract
- 1/8 tsp cinnamon

INGREDIENTS: TOPPINGS

- 1/2 medium seeded pomegranate
- 1 sliced banana
- 2 chopped roughly dates
- 1-2 Tbsp sunflower seeds
- 1-2 Tbsp pumpkin seeds

DIRECTIONS

Mix all puding ingredients until combined. Let them sit for 10 minutes, and then mix again to avoid clumping.

Cover and put in the fridge for 1 to 2 hours, or you can leave it overnight.

Mix well before serving, pour it into a bowl and add the desired toppings. I used bananas, pomegranate seeds, pumpkin seeds and sunflower seeds, but use your imagination and feel free to add the fruits and nuts you desire.

8. Plantain Pancakes

Servings: 2

Preparation time: 15 min

Cooking time: 20 minutes

Ingredients

- 1 large ripe banana plantains
- 1 cup all purpose flour
- 3/4 cup unsweetened plant-based milk
- 1 cup all purpose flour
- 1/2 tsp vanilla
- 2 tsp coconut oil
- Oil for frying (coconut or grapeseed oil)
- 1 tbsp Pure Maple Syrup
- 1 1/2 teaspoons baking powder

Optional:

1 tsp cinnamon

Fruit: strawberries, blueberries, raspberries

Brown sugar

Instructions

Mash the peeled banana in a bowl, and add the plant-based milk, vanilla, maple syrup and coconut oil. Whisk it quickly, and add the flour and baking powder. Whisk until all ingredients are incorporated.

On a medium heat, put the oil in a flat pan. Once heated, add part of the pancake batter. Once you notice that the middle is becoming bubbly, flip it with a spatula, and leave it to cook on the other side. Repeat the same process for the other pancakes. Usually I am able to make around 6 pancakes out of the batter.

Top the pancakes with maple syrup and the desired fruit. Enjoy!

Lunch:

9. Spaghetti Squash with Veggie Tomato Sauce

Servings: 4

Preparation time: 1 hour

Ingredients:

- 1 large Spaghetti Squash
- 2 canned crushed tomatoes
- 2 cups of already cooked lentils
- 1 tsp dried basil
- 1 1/2 tsps Olive Oil
- 1 minced Garlic clove
- 1/4 tsp Sea Salt
- 1/4 tsp Black Pepper
- 4 cups Baby Spinach (chopped)
- 1/2 cup Hemp Seeds

Optional:

For more veggies: diced

- Zucchini
- Mushrooms
- Eggplants
- To the sauce

1. Preheat the oven to 400 degrees F. Start with the spaghetti squash. Cut them on half and take out the seeds.

2. On a baking sheet with parchment paper, place the two halves, and add olive oil, sea salt and a bit of paper. Turn the squash flesh side down and put it in the oven for 40 minutes.

3. Meanwhile, combine the crushed tomatoes, lentils, garlic, the dried basil, sea salt, black pepper, dried basil in a pot over medium heat and bring it to simmer. Once ready, add the spinach and mux until wilted.

4. When the spaghetti squash is ready, take it out from the oven and let it cool. Carve out the flesh into noodles so that the liquid can drain off.

5. Put the spaghetti squash in a bowl for serving. Add a spoon of the vegetable tomato sauce over the top and enjoy!

10. Creamy Mushroom Pasta

Servings: 4

Preparation time: 10 minutes

Cooking time: 20 minutes

Ingredients:

- 400g fusilli or some other type of pasta if preferred
- 10 mL vegetable oil
- 2 large shallots
- 6 cloves garlic
- 1 fresh red chili
- 500 mL vegetable broth
- 1 can or 400 ml coconut milk
- 400 g mushrooms
- 30 g sun-dried tomato
- 100g spinach
- 10 g nutritional yeast
- 15 mL sodium-reduced soy sauce
- 4 g ground paprika
- Pepper and salt to taste

Optional:

Basil

Chili flakes

On a high heat, for 3 minutes, sautè the minced garlic, the finely chopped onions and the minced chili. Add the sun dried tomato and the mushrooms.

Add the broth, and the coconut oil. Bring to boil, and add the pasta. Reduce to simmer and stir occasionally.

Once the pasta is ready, the cooking time depends on the type of pasta and usually is indicated on the package, preferably choosing pasta with 10 – 12 minutes cooking time. Once ready remove it from the heat, and add the spinach.

Mix to combine.

Add some basil leaves, chilli flakes, and squeeze some fresh lemon juice.

Enjoy it while hot!

Notes

Storage: You can make this dish also as meal prep and keep it in fridge, in an air-tight container, for up to 2 days.

11. Mung Bean Soup

Servings: 3-4

Preparation time: 10 minutes

Cooking times: 25 minutes

INGREDIENTS

- 1 cup dried mung bean soaked overnight/6 hours, drain and rinsed
- 1 chopped onion
- 3 minced garlic gloves
- 1 chopped carrot
- 14oz can diced tomatoes
- 4 cups water
- 1 cup coconut milk
- 3 tbsp avocado oil

Spices

- 1/2 tsp Turmeric
- 1/2 tsp curry powder
- 1/2 tsp ground cumin
- 1/2 tsp ginger ground
- 1/2 tsp garam masala
- 1/2 tsp brown mustard seeds
- pinch of cayenne pepper
- 1 tsp salt
- pepper to taste

Optional:

fresh herbs

INSTRUCTIONS

1. In a medium pot add the onions and saute together with the garlic. Once the onion is soft, add the carrots, and continue to stir for 3-4 minutes.
2. Add the tomatoes, spices, salt and pepper. Mix for another 5 minutes.
3. Add the mung beans, and mix for another 2 minutes.
4. Add water, bring it to boil and let it simmer for another 20 minutes. You will note that it is ready when the mung beans will become tender.
5. Add coconut milk and let it simmer for another 10 minutes.
6. Serve it in a bowl. Enjoy!

12. Mashed Chickpea & Dill Sandwich

Serving: 3-4 sandwiches

Preparation Time: 10 minutes

Total Time: 10 minutes

INGREDIENTS
- 4 slices of toasted whole wheat bread, toasted
- 250 g cooked chickpeas
- 1/2 finely chopped bell pepper
- 1/4 finely chopped red onion
- 35 g finely chopped dill pickle
- 60 ml vegan mayo or tahini
- 30 g roasted sunflower seeds
- 2 Tbsp fresh dill, coarsely chopped or 1 Tbsp of dried chili
- 1-2 leaves of fresh lettuce

Optional:
1 Tbsp chopped fresh chives
Basil
Cumin

Directions
1. In a large bowl add and mash the chickpeas with a fork until they get flakey.
2. Add the bell pepper, pickles, red onion, sunflower seeds, vegan mayo, dill and chives. Mix until all ingredients are combined.
3. You can serve it on a toasted bread and lettuce, on a salad, in a wrap, or as a delicious dip for crackers and vegetables.

Notes:

If you want to accelerate the process you can use canned beans. If switching for canned chickpeas, this is the amount in a 500 g can. You need to rinse them first and as they are higher in salt, taste, and add the salt at the end.
You can store it for up to 2 days in an air-tight container in the fridge.

13. Spicy Garlic Wok Noodles with Stir-fried Veg & Tofu

Serving: 3-4 portions

Preparation Time: 15 minutes

Cooking Time: 25 minutes

INGREDIENTS

- 250 g sliced mushrooms
- 15 mL oil
- 180g seasoned tofu strips
- 4 crushed garlic cloves
- 1 finely chopped red onion
- 1/4 tsp ground black pepper
- 120 g wok noodles
- 1 thinly sliced carrot
- Half large head of broccoli, cut to florets
- 2 red bell peppers, cut into thin strips
- 2 Tbsp sambal (or chili paste)
- 2 Tbsp ketjap (or Indonesian sweet soy sauce)
- 1 Tbsp soy sauce (tamari if GF)

Optional:
- 2 Tbsp roasted sesame seeds for garnish
- Fresh chili
- Quinoa or rice instead of noodles

Directions
1. In a large pot on a high heat, put the oil and mushrooms. Reduce the heat to medium after 5 minutes, and stir on

occasion until the water from the mushrooms begins to evaporate.

2. While this cooks, chop the vegetables.
3. Increase the heat to high, and add the tofu, onion, garlic and black pepper. Mix frequently for about 5 minutes, until the garlic gets brown and the onion becomes transparent.
4. In the meantime, prepare the wok noodle. Check the instructions and cook it accordingly until al dente.
5. Add the vegetables to the pot and leave it to cook for another 5 minutes.
6. Add the soy sauce, sambal and ketjap and cook for another 2 minutes.
7. Mix it together and cook for few more minutes. Add the already cooked noodles also and mix again until well combined.
8. Decorate with sesame seeds and fresh chilli. Serve while hot.

Notes:

You can prepare the dish during meal prep and store it in the fridge for up to three days.

14. Bean & Oat Burger with 3-ingredient Cajun Mayo

Servings: 4 - 6 patties

Preparation Time: 15 minutes

Cooking Time: 25 minutes

INGREDIENTS: Burger Patty

- 115g rolled oats, or breadcrumbs
- 15g ground flax seeds
- 1 finely diced yellow onion
- 2 crushed garlic cloves
- 400g cooked pinto beans
- 50g sunflower seeds or walnuts (either raw or roasted)
- 5mL olive oil
- 5g ground cumin
- 5g paprika powder
- 5g cajun seasoning spice

INGREDIENTS: Accompaniments

- 4-6 burger buns
- 440g thinly sliced button mushrooms
- 2 thinly sliced medium red bell peppers
- 5mL olive oil
- 1/2 tsp onion powder
- 1/2 tsp garlic powder
- 1/2 tsp cumin
- 1/2 tsp paprika

- 30g arugula, or other leafy green if you prefer

Optional:
20g raw or pickled jalapeño slices

INGREDIENTS: Cajun Mayo
- 50g raw cashews, soaked in water for 50-60 minutes
- 1 juiced lime
- 8g cajun seasoning spice

Directions

1. In a food processor add 6 tbsp of water together with the ground flax seeds. Let it sit for 5-7 minutes until the flax seeds gel.
2. On high heat fry the onions with oil on a medium pan, for 5 minutes. Add splashes of water in order to prevent it from burning. Add the garlic and sauté for another 2 minutes.
3. Once ready, add them to the food processor, together with the remaining ingredients. Blend on a high temperature well until combined.
4. Prepare the rest of the ingredients: fry the mushrooms in oil and after 5 minutes add the bell pepper and spices. Cook for another 3 minutes, and if necessary add a bit of water to prevent it from burning.
5. To prepare the Cajun mayo, in a blender, blend all ingredients with ¼ cup water.
6. From the patties from the bean and oat mixture. Cook them on

a non-stick pan together with 1/2 tsp oil per patty per side. It will need 3 to 4 minutes per side.

7. Arrange the burger buns with the patties, arugula, sautéed mushroom and bell pepper, cajun mayo and jalapeños. Enjoy!

8. You can store the patties up to 3 days in the fridge, and up to 2 months in a freezer.

15. Tomato Lentil Pasta

Servings: 4-5

Preparation Time: 10 minutes

Cook Time: 20 minutes

INGREDIENTS

- 15 mL vegetable oil
- chopped onion
- 4 minced garlic gloves
- 1 vegetable bouillon cube
- 1 tsp Italian seasoning mix (or basil or sub dried oregano)
- ½ tsp red chili pepper flakes
- 300 g dry spaghetti
- 750 mL pasta sauce
- 300 g halved cherry tomatoes
- 300 g cooked brown lentils
- 50 g sliced or chopped black olives
- 25 g chopped sun-dried tomatoes
- 10 g capers
- 60 g fresh spinach

Optional
Thinly sliced

Directions

1. In a large pot on medium-high heat the oil and add the onion,

garlic, bouillon cube, Italian seasoning, and the red chili pepper flakes. Fry it for 3 minutes and add splashes of water to deglaze the pot.

2. Pour the water to the pot and bring it to boil. Add the pasta, pasta sauce, lentils, cherry tomatoes, olives, sun-dried tomatoes, and capers. Bring to a gentle simmer and cover partially with a lid. Cook for 10-15 minutes, depending of the type of pasta. Check on the package. Stir it occasionally to ensure that   nothing sticks to the bottom of the pot.

3. When the pasta is al dente, add the spinach and mix.

4. Serve it with some freshly sliced basil leaves as decoration. Enjoy!

5. You can keep it in an air-tight container in the fridge for up to 3 days.

Snacks:

16. Green Boost Juice

Servings: 1

Preparation time: 5 minutes

Ingredients:

- cup Baby Spinach
- Persian Cucumber
- 1/2 cup frozen Pineapple
- 1/4 Avocado
- cups filtered water
- 1/4 cup Vanilla Protein Powder
- tbsp peeled Ginger
- 1 tbsp Sunflower Seeds
- 1 tbsp Lemon Juice

Optional

1 tsp of spirulina or chlorella

Place all ingredients in the blender and pulse until smooth. Pour into a glass and enjoy!

17. The Violet Smoothie

Servings: 2

Preparation Time: 5 minutes

INGREDIENTS
- 500 mL plant-based milk
- 100 g frozen blueberries
- 2 ripe and frozen bananas
- 5 mL pure vanilla extract
- 30 mL almond butter

Optional:
Whole almonds
Spinach
Strawberries

DIRECTIONS

Blend all ingredients together until well combined. Add the desired toppings and enjoy immediately.

18. Pumpkin Flax Seed Bombs

Servings: 11

Preparation times: 10 minutes

Ingredients:

- 32g Almond Butter
- 32g Ground Flax Seed
- 32g Pumpkin Seeds
- 64g cup Cashews
- 64g cup Unsweetened Coconut Flakes
- 32g Cacao Nibs
- 32g Coconut Oil
- 64g cup Pitted Dates (4 Dates)
    - tsp Cinnamon
- 1/2 tsp Vanilla Extract

Optional:

scoop of collagen peptides

1. Put together all ingredients in a food processor or blender. Blend until roughly combined and begins to form a dough.
2. Roll the paste into balls and lay flat into an airtight container. Pay attention the balls to not touch each other, as they will stick together
3. It can be kept in the freezer for 3 to 4 months.

19. Easy Guacamole Recipe

Preparation time: 10 minutes

INGREDIENTS

- 4 ripe avocados
- handful fresh cilantro
- 2 limes
- 2 tbsp olive oil
- sea salt and pepper to taste
- Optional: 1 small onion

INSTRUCTIONS

1. Cut avocados in half, peel skin and remove core. Cut them into small cubes and put them in a mixing bowl.
2. Mash the avocados with fork or a potato masher.
3. Add to the bowl the finely diced onion.
4. Next, chop finely and add also the cilantro to the bowl.
5. Squeeze the juice from the 2 limes into the bowl.
6. Add sea salt and pepper to taste.
7. Add 2 tbsp of olive oil.
8. Mix all together. Serve it with some cilantro on the top!

In case your avocados are not mature enough, just place them in a brown paper bag and add banana or apple. The brown bag together with the added fruit will increase the emission of the ethylene gas and keep it in inside the bag, which will lead to speed up the ripening process.

20. Sweet Sesame Balls

Preparation time: 10 minutes

Servings: 12 balls

INGREDIENTS

- 7 Medjool Dates
- 1/2 cup Pumpkin Seeds
- 1/2 cup Sunflower Seeds
- 1/4 cup Sesame Butter/Tahini
- 3 tbsp Cocoa powder
- pinch Sea salt

INSTRUCTIONS

- Place all ingredients into a food processor.
- Pulse until the seeds are finely chopped and well combined.
- Take the mixture and with the hands form small round balls.
- Enjoy!

21. Zucchini Fries with dip

Servings: 3 - 4

Preparation Time: 10 minutes

Cook Time: 30 minutes

INGREDIENTS

- 2 medium zucchini
- 85 g breadcrumbs
- 10 mL vegetable oil
- 2 Tbsp nutritional yeast
- tsp salt
- ½ tsp ground black pepper

Roasted Red Pepper Dip

- 2 roasted red bell peppers from a jar
- 5 mL sambal oelek
- ½ tsp garlic powder
- ½ tsp dried oregano
- ½ tsp dried basil

Directions

1. Preheat the oven to 340°F/170°C. Cut the zucchini into 1 inch thick fries, and put them in a large shallow bowl.
2. Toss the zucchini with oil. Add the nutritional yeast, breadcrumbs, salt and pepper. Mix well to coat the zucchini. Put the zucchini into a parchment lined baking dish.
3. Bake for 20 minutes. Flip the zucchini to help it cook evenly, and then leave it in the oven for another 15 - 20 minutes. You will note that they are ready when they will get soft on the inside, and

golden on the outside.

4. To make the dip, add all ingredients in a food processor, and blend until coarsely chopped.

5. You can store it in a container, preferably air-tight container, in the fridge for up to 3 days.

22. Green and Black olives tapenade

Serving: approx. 1.5 cups

Preparation Time: **15 min**

INGREDIENTS
- 200g pitted kalamata olives
- 200g pitted green olives
- 30g sun-dried tomatoes
- 1og capers
- 2 garlic cloves
- 2g chopped fresh basil
- 5g dried oregano
- 15mL olive oil
- 30mL lemon juice, about 1/2 a lemon

Optional:
45g roasted walnuts

Directions

1. In a medium bow put the finely minced olives, capers, sun-dried tomatoes, garli , basil and walnuts.
2. Add the rest of the ingredients and mix to combine.
3. Decorate with fresh basil. You can enjoy it immediately, but I advise you to cover it and put it in the fridge for 2 hours or overnight to allow flavours to meld.
1. You can store it in an air-tight container in the fridge for up to two weeks.

23. La Macedonia

Serving: approx. 4 cups

Preparation Time: 10 minutes

Total Time: 10 min

INGREDIENTS: Fruit Salad
- peeled and cubed mango
- cubed kiwis
- 150g fresh blueberries
- 75 g fresh strawberries, quartered
- 150g purple grapes

INGREDIENTS: Sweet Lime Dressing
- 1/2 lime, juice and zest
- Optional: 5 mL agave syrup

Directions

1. Add all fruit to a large bowl.
2. Mix together the agave syrup with the lime juice in a small bowl. Add it to the fruit and mix well.
1. Store the salad in an air-tight container in the fridge for up to one day. It is better if you can store the dressing separately.

Dessert:

24. Raspberry and Rhubarb Almond Tart

Servings: 6-8

Preparation time: 15 minutes

Cooking time: 30 minutes

Ingredients

For the crust:

- 155 g roasted almonds, with skin
- 3 soft dates, pitted
- 30 ml coconut oil
- 15 g buckwheat flour
- 5 ml vanilla

For the filling:

- 125 g roasted almonds, with skin
- 100g sugar
- 125 ml vegan margarine
- 40 g plain flour
- 90 ml water
- 21 g ground flaxseed
- 50 g fresh raspberries

- 60 g fresh rhubarb, washed, peeled and cut into 1 inch pieces

1. In a food processor, blend together all the ingredients for the crust: the buckwheat flour, almonds, the dates and the vanilla until you get a sand-like density. Melt also the coconut oil and add to the mixture. Mix it together with the rest of the ingredients.
2. Transfer the mix to a parchment lined tart tray and using your fingers press the mixture into the tray.
3. Preheat the oven at 180 C (350 F).
4. The next step is to prepare the filling. Combine the flaxseed with water and leave them aside to gel. In the meantime, in the food processor again, combine together the almonds, the vegan margarine, sugar and flour. Mix it until you get a paste, and add the flaxseed mixture. Mix again.
5. Transfer the filling into the prepared crust.
6. Wash the raspberries and the rhubarb. Peel the rhubarb and cut it on 1 inch pieces.
7. Decorate the tart with the freshed raspberries and the chopped rhubarb.
8. Into the oven it goes for 30 minutes. When you note that the crust starts to golden at the edges it means it's ready.
9. Wait to cool. If you wish, decorate it with a bit of powdered sugar.

Tip: It can be conserved in the fridge for up to 6-7 days.

Do not forget to let me know in the comments if you make some of the recipes and if you liked them. And I am especially curious about this one!

25. Lemon Cups

Servings: 24

Preparation time: 15 minutes

Cooking time: 60 minutes

Ingredients:

For the base:

- 45 g raw almonds
- 40 g raw walnuts
- 50 g shredded coconuts, unsweetened
- 12 soft medjool dates
- 1/8 tsp salt

The filling:

- 225 g raw cashews
- 8 soft medjool dates
- 5 lemons, (we need the juice of two and the zest of one lemon.)
- 1/2 tsp pure vanilla extract

Directions:

01. If possible, soak the nuts previously. Even 10 minutes are enough, but you can soak them as well for a few hours.
02. In the food processor, blend together the almonds and the walnuts until you get flour.

03. Add the dates, shredded coconuts, the dates and the salt and blend for a few more minutes to combine all ingredients.

04. With a teaspoon add part of the mixture in a 24-cup mini muffin pan. Press down gently.

05. Once ready, place the muffin pan in the freezer.

06. Prepare the cream filling. Blend together all ingredients for the filling in a food processor: the cashews, the lemon zest and the lemon juice, the dates and the vanilla extract. In case the dates are not soft, soak them in water for 10 minutes. Blend all until you get a soft cream.

07. Add the cream on the top of each muffin base, and sprinkle the shredded coconut.

08. Let them cool in the freezer for 1 hour.

09. Once ready, use a butter knife around the edge to take the cups out.

Keep the muffins in the freezer until serving.

26. Cranberry Lime Balls

Servings: 24 servings

Preparation time: 20 minutes

Ingredients:

- 90g dried cranberries
- 140 g raw almonds
- 150 g raw cashews
- 1/8 tsp salt
- 175 g dates
- 2 limes, juice and zest
- 75 g unsweetened shredded coconut
- 90 g dried cranberries

1. Blend the cashews, almonds and salt In a food processor. Put them aside in a large mixing bowl.
2. Combine the dates, the lime juice, lime zest and the shredded coconut in the food processor. Blend until you get a soft paste.
3. Once ready, add the date paste to the nut flour in the bowl. Add the dried cranberries and mix.
4. Using your hand form small balls from the mixture.
5. Roll the balls in diverse toppings: shredded coconut, lime zest or chopped dried cranberries.
   Keep them in the fridge or the freezer!

27. Homemade Dark Chocolate Date Turtles

Servings: 25

Preparation time: 25 minutes

INGREDIENTS

- 80 pecan halves
- 7 medjool dates
- 2 tsp vanilla extract
- salt to sprinkle
- Camino chocolate bar
- a bit of water

INSTRUCTIONS

1. In a food processor combine the pitted dates together with the vanilla. Add a bit of water to make it smooth as caramel.
2. Make the date paste into small balls and place it on parchment paper. Add 3 pecans to each date ball.
3. Decora with melted chocolate on the top and add salt if you want. Personally I prefer sea salt on some occasions, while in others I avoid to add it.
4. Keep in the fridge until the chocolate hardens. Enjoy!

28. Homemade Paleo Dark Chocolate

Servings: 15, but it depends of the molds

Preparing time: 5-10 minutes

Ingredients:

- 105g coconut oil
- 120g cocoa powder
- Pinch of sea salt
- Optional:
- Vanilla extract
- Nut butter
- Honey
- Almonds
- Mint
- Blueberries and cranberries
- Banana
- Chilli powder

Preparation:

01. Melt the coconut oil on a low heat, in a small pot.
02. Once melted, remove it from the heat and add the cocoa powder, sea salt and any other other ingredients you want. Mix everything together.
03. Put the mixture into silicone molds and put in the fridge for one year.
04. Once hardened, pop them out of the molds and enjoy!

Tip: In case you wish to add honey, I recommend to put the mixture in the fridge for a few minutes before adding it. In this way, as the honey is heavier, it will not stay on the bottom of the pot.

I love this recipe. It can be made in no time, and it can be used as a base, and can be personalized depending on your preferences.

29. Easy Chocolate Cake

Servings: 12

Preparation Time: 30 minutes

Cooking Time: 30 minutes

INGREDIENTS: Cake
- 240 mL unsweetened plant-based milk
- 15 mL white vinegar
- 240 g all purpose flour
- 315 g granulated sugar
- 100 g cacao powder
- 1½ tsp baking soda
- 2 tsp or 8 g baking powder
- ½ tsp salt
- 240 mL unsweetened applesauce
- 120 mL freshly brewed espresso
- 120 mL melted coconut oil
- 8 mL pure vanilla extract
- 5 mL melted coconut oil
- 4 g all purpose flour

INGREDIENTS: Frosting
- 225g soften unsalted plant-based butter
- 50 g cacao powder
- 5 mL vanilla extract
- 240 g powdered sugar
- 60 mL unsweetened plant-based milk
- 60 mL melted dairy-free dark chocolate

Decorations
Strawberries
Blackberries
Raspberries
Blueberries
Mint leaves
 Nuts

DIRECTIONS

1. Preheat the oven to 350°F/180°C. Start making the vegan buttermilk.Mix the milk together with the vinegar. You will note it starts to curdle.
2. Sift all dry ingredients in a large bowl, and mix them together.
3. Add the buttermilk and the rest of the wet ingredients. Mix all together until there are no lumps left, but be careful to not over mix it.
4. Grease with oil two 8-inch round cake pans, and put a piece of cut-out round parchment paper on the bottom.
5. Divide the cake batter into the two cake pans and bake them for 30 - 35 minutes.
6. In the meantime, start making the frosting. In a large bowl, sift the cacao powder, ass the butter and the vanilla, and mix with a hand mixer, or an electric one, until you get smooth and creamy consistency.
7. Alternate between adding plant-based milk and sifted powdered sugar in the bowl, until all ingredients are well combined.
8. Fold in the melted chocolate and make sure to let it cool off a little bit before adding.
9. Once the cakes finished baking and are ready, let them cool off for 15-20 minutes in the cake pan, before transferring them on a cooling rack to let them cool off completely.
10. If you prefer, you can level your cakes with a serrated knife, in

order to create a flat surface to be able to stack the cakes on top of each other.

11. With a butter knife or a spatula, lay out a thick layer of frosting on one of the cakes. Put the second cake on top of it and frost with the leftover frosting. If you like you can even create a pattern.

12. Decorate the chocolate cake with fruit of your choice, nuts if you desire and some mint leaves. Enjoy!

13. The cake can be stored in the fridge for up to 3 days.

30. Homemade Nutella

Serving: approx. 1.5 cups

Prep Time: 10 min

Cook Time: 10 min

INGREDIENTS

- 225 g raw hazelnuts
- 80 mL unsweetened plant milk. I used homemade avena milk.
- 6 soft dates
- 35 g coconut powder
- 15 mL coconut oil
- 30 mL maple
- 5 mL vanilla extract
- ¼ tsp salt

Directions

1. Preheat the oven to 350 F/ 180 C. Bake the hazelnuts for 10-12 minutes, until fragrant and lightly golden, stir it occasionally. Once ready, remove from the oven. Let it cool for a while!
2. Rub firmly between your palms or rub them with a kitchen cloth so the skin falls off.
3. Put the hazelnuts in a food processor or a high-speed blender. Blend on high for 5 minutes, or until you get nut butter consistency.
4. Add the rest of the ingredients and blend again for an additional 4-5 minutes until all ingredients are well incorporated and you get smooth butter.
5. It can be stored in an air-tight container in the fridge for up to 7 days.

31. Choc chunk and zucchini bread

Ingredients:

- 1/2 cup almond flour
- 1/3 cup coconut flour
- cup organic shredded zucchini
- 1/2 cup dark choc (75-90% cacao), chopped into chunks
- 1/3 organic coconut sugar
- 4 flax eggs
- 1/2 cup liquid coconut oil
- teaspoons baking powder
- 1/2 teaspoon vanilla essence
- teaspoon cinnamon
- (make sure you really squeeze out all the moisture!)
- Extra dark choc chunks to decorate on top
- Pinch of salt

DIRECTIONS

Preheat the oven to 350 degrees. Grease the bread dish well, or line it with parchment paper .

Mix the eggs with the coconut sugar, coconut oil and the vanilla.

Add in the almond flour, coconut flour and baking powder .Mix until all ingredients are well combined

Squeeze out all the moisture from the zucchini. Add the zucchini, pinch of salt, and then the dark chocolate hunks to the rest of the ingredients.

Top with some extra choc and bake it in the oven for 45-50 minutes. Enjoy!

It can be stored in the fridge for 5 days or in the freezer for a couple of months.

Dinner:

32. Eggplant and lentil curry

Servings: 3

Preparation time: 5 minutes

Cook time: 20 minutes

Ingredients:

- 2 eggplants
- diced onion
- garlic cloves
- bell red pepper
- can (400 mL) of diced tomatoes
- 265 g cooked brown lentils
- 30 g dried apricots
- 8g ground cumin
- 4g ground cinnamon
- 8g coriander
- 5ml olive oil
- 10 ml coconut oil
- 4g salt
- ½ tsp salt
- ¼ tsp ground black pepper

Optional:

Lemon wedges

Fresh mint leaves, thinly sliced

Coconut yogurt

01. Turn on the oven to 200°C (400°F). Start preparing the eggplants. Cut the tops off, each of them cut in half lengthwise. Cut cross-hatches into the flesh of each half. Sprinkle some oil and salt on each half, and rub in.
02. Prepare a parchment lined baking sheet and bake them for 20 minutes. Use a fork to check them if ready.
03. Let them cool, and once ready, scrape out the cooked part with a spoon and set it aside.
04. In a large pot heat the coconut oil in a medium heat and sauté the minced onion for 5 minutes. If needed add some water.
05. Add the minced garlic, cinnamon, cumin and coriander. Sauté for another minute.
06. Add the diced bell pepper, can of tomatoes, the brown lentils , the dried apricots and the roasted eggplant. Finally, add the salt and pepper and heat until the peppers become crunchy and soft.
07. Add some coconut yogurt or fresh lemon if you want. Enjoy the curry with naan or some rice. The white rice you can substitute with the brown.

33. Rainbow salad

Servings: 4-6

Preparation time:10 time

Cooking time: 20 minutes

Ingredients:

Salade:

- 370g cooked quinoa
- 165g cooked chickpeas
- 30g dried cranberries
- 2 red bell peppers (we used 1 red and 1 yellow)
- medium-sized tomato, seeded and chopped
- 1/3 cucumber, diced
- 13-15 kalamata olives, pitted and chopped
- sprig green onion, thinly sliced
- 70g roasted almonds, coarsely chopped

Dressing:

- 2 lemons, juiced
- (30 mL olive oil
- head of garlic (about 8 cloves)
- 15 mL tahini
- 5 mL sodium-reduced soy sauce
- 5 mL balsamic vinegar
- tsp onion powder

- Salt and pepper to taste

DIRECTIONS

Turn on the oven to Preheat at 200 C/390 F.

Take the garlic and cut the top off it. Put it on a baking sheet, drizzle it with a bit of olive oil and put it in the oven for 15 minutes. You will note that it will get golden once ready.

In the meantime, cut all vegetables. Put them in a large bowl together with the chickpeas, the cooked quinoa and the cranberries.

Mash the garlic with a fork and add it to the rest of the ingredients. Mix to combine.

Put the dressing over the salad and toss to combine. Decorate with the toasted almonds and enjoy!

34. Budha Tempeh Bowl

Servings: 2

Preparation time: 30 minutes

Ingredients:

- 6 ozs Tempeh, sliced into strips
- 2 2/3 cups Cauliflower Rice
- 4 cups Arugula
- 1/3 tbsps Tamari
- tsps Avocado Oil
- 1/8 tsp Paprika
- 1/3 tbsps Lemon Juice
- tbsps Tahini
- tsps Maple Syrup
- tbsps Water
- 1/16 tsp Sea Salt
- 2/3 sliced Avocado
- 2 tbsps Sunflower Seeds

Optional:

Chili

Cooked sweet potato

1. Preheat the oven to 375°F/191°C. Toss the tempeh with the avocado oil, paprika and tamari, and place it on a baking sheet with parchment paper. Bake for 10 minutes each side.
2. On a frying pan put the riced cauliflower. Sauté for 5 to 7 minutes.
3. In a small bowl, whisk together the tahini, water, maple syrup, lemon juice and sea salt.
4. Put the cauliflower rice to a serving bowl, and top with avocado, arugula, tempeh and sunflower seeds. Add the tahini dressing and enjoy!
5. It can be kept in a fridge in an air-tight container up to 3 days.

35. Yucca Pizza Dough

Servings: 2

Preparation Time: 20 minutes

Cook time: 15 minutes

Ingredients:

- 20g coconut flour
- 250g cubed yucca
- 65g Extra Virgin Olive Oil
- 2.5g garlic salt
- 2.5g baking powder

For the toppings:

- Tomato sauce
- Mushrooms
- peppers
- zucchini
- zucchini, mushrooms, peppers
- nutritional yeast

INSTRUCTIONS

1. Firstly, preheat the oven.
2. Peel the yucca, cut it into cubes dand boil it for around 15 minutes. Check with a fork when it's ready.
3. In a food processor, blend the yucca together with the olive

oil, scraping the sides as needed. Blend until it starts to form a ball of dough.

4. In another bowl, sift the coconut flour. Add in the baking powder and garlic salt.

5. Add the dry ingredients to the mashed yucca.

6. Place the dough on a baking sheet and with the help of a piece of parchment paper, flatten the dough until it becomes 1/8 inch thick.

7. Remove the parchment paper and put the dough in the oven for 20 minutes or until it gets golden brown.

8. Once ready, add the tomato sauce and the toppings.

9. Get it back in the oven and cook for a few more minutes until the toppings are cooked.

36. The Roasted Soup

Servings: 4

Preparation time: 5 minutes

Cooking time: 30 minutes

Ingredients:

- ½ butternut squash, peeled and cut into 2 cm 1 inch chunks, seeds reserved
- 2 bell peppers, de-seeded and cut into quarters
- sliced red onion
- jalapeño, de-seeded and cut in half
- carrots, cut into 2 cm pieces
- 6 peeled cloves of garlic
- 200 mL coconut milk
- 750 mL vegetable stock
- tsp olive oil
- ½ tsp salt
- ½ tsp pepper
- ½ tsp paprika powder
- ½ tsp ground cumin
- Roasted Squash Seeds
- Squash seeds
- 1 tsp (5 mL) olive oil
- ¼ tsp paprika powder
- ¼ tsp garlic powder
- ¼ tsp onion powder
- ¼ tsp salt

- ¼ tsp ground cumin
- ¼ tsp fresh ground pepper

Directions

On a baking sheet toss all the vegetables with spices and olive oil, and cook for 30 minutes at 350°F/180°C. Check with a fork if the squash and the carrots are tender.

In the meantime, clean off the butternut squash seeds, toss with spices and oil. Place it in another baking sheet and put it in the oven for 15 minutes or until they get crunchy and golden. Toss 1-2 times while they are cooking.

Once the vegetables are ready, put them in a large pot on high heat together with the coconut milk vegetable stock. Blend them with an immersion blender.

Once ready, reheat it, and top with roasted squash seed and coconut cream.

It can be kept in the fridge in an air-tight container for up to 3 days.

37. Sweet potato and beetroot soup

Servings: 5-6 servings

Preparation Time: 10 minutes

Cook Time: 30 minutes

INGREDIENTS:

- 2 beetroots, peeled and cut in 1 cm chunks
- 3 sweet potatoes, peeled and cut into 1 cm chunks
- 2 chopped yellow onions
- 2 crushed garlic cloves garlic
- 400 mL full fat coconut milk
- 5 mL olive oil
- vegetable bouillon cube
- tsp cumin powder
- 1/2 tsp paprika powder

Optional:

Pumpkin seeds

Coconut milk

Fresh herbs

In a large pot on a high heat, add the oil and onions for 5-7 minutes, or until the onions caramelize. Add a bit of water as needed to deglaze the pan. Once ready, add the garlic and stir for 2 minutes, until it becomes.

Pour 2 cups of water and except for the coconut milk, add all the remaining ingredients to the pot. Bring to a boil, then reduce to a simmer with the lid partially covering.

Once the beetroots and the potatoes are soft, puree completely using a standing or immersion blender.

Get the soup back on low heat, and add the coconut milk, stirring to combine. Put the lid and allow the soup to warm back up, about 2 minutes.

Once ready, it can be served. Top with coconut milk, fresh herbs or pumpkin seeds.

It can be stored in an air-tight container in the fridge for up to four days. In the freezer it can be stored for up to two months.

38. Focaccia Pizza

Yield: 2 servings

Preparation Time: 10 minutes

Cooking Time: 20 minutes

INGREDIENTS

- 500 g can tomato sauce
- 68 g tin tomato puree
- 3 crushed cloves garlic
- 10g dried oregano
- 15g nutritional yeast
- 5g Italian spice mix, or sub dried basil
- 1/2 tsp curry powder
- freshly ground pepper
- thinly sliced red bell pepper
- 5 thinly sliced large mushrooms, thinly sliced
- 1/2 thinly sliced red onion
- 10 cherry tomatoes, cut in half
- 20 kalamata olives, cut in half
- 30g fresh arugula

INGREDIENTS: Tahini Balsamic Sauce

- 30ml tahini
- 10ml balsamic vinegar

Optional:

Any other veggies you like:

- zucchini

 - spinach

- green olives, etc.

Directions

Preheat the oven to 350 F/180C. Cut the focaccia bread in half and place it on a cooking sheet.

Mix together the tomato puree concentrate with pepper until well combined. Spread this pizza sauce on the bread. Add the vegetables on the top, and place in the oven for about 20 minutes.

In the meantime, prepare the drizzle. Mix together the tahini with balsamic vinegar, and add 2 Tbsp of water. Mix until creamy and well combined.

When the pizza is ready, remove from the oven, drizzle on the tahini balsamic sauce and add with the fresh arugula.

39. Autumn Magic Nourish Bowl

Servings: 4-5

Preparation Time: 10 minutes

Cooking Time: 50 minutes

INGREDIENTS: The Bowl

- 260 g dry quinoa, rinsed
- 1.5L vegetable broth or 1 vegetable bouillon cube
- thinly sliced red onion
- minced garlic gloves
- 350 g Brussels sprouts
- sweet potatoes, cut into 2cm cubes
- 15 mL vegetable or olive oil
- 60 g leafy greens of choice
- 45 g coarsely chopped roasted almonds, coarsely chopped
- 45 g pomegranate seeds
- 15 g dried cranberries

INGREDIENTS: The Sauce

- 60mL tahini
- 45mL water
- tsp miso paste, or soy sauce
- tsp dijon mustard
- 1/2 tsp turmeric powder
- 1/2 juiced lemon
- 1/2 tsp onion powder

- freshly cracked black pepper

Optional ingredients:

- red bell peppers

- zucchini.

- hummus

Directions

Preheat the oven to 220 C/425 F

Spread the onion, garlic, sweet potatoes and Brussels sprouts with oil, in a baking dish. Stir occasionally. Cook about 50 minutes or until cooked to your liking.

Put the quinoa in a pot with 560 mL water and crush in the bouillon cube. Bring to boil and reduce the heat to low. Cover partially, and leave it to cook for around 2 minutes, until the liquid is absorbed and the quinoa is al dente.

In a food processor add the sauce ingredients and blend until well combined. Or you can mix them in a bowl instead.

To create the Autumn Magic Nourish bowl, combine the quinoa, greens and baked veggies. Top with almonds, cranberries and pomegranate seeds. Drizzle the sauce and enjoy!

Store in an air-tight container in the fridge for up to four days. Store the sauce separately for up to 3 days.

40. Vegan broccoli, cauliflower and leek immune boosting soup

Servings: 4-6

Ingredients:

- large broccoli
- 2 heads of cauliflower
- peeled and chopped potatoes
- chopped onion
- 4 crushed garlic
- Litre of vegetable broth
- can of coconut milk
- -3 Tbsp extra virgin olive oil
- 4 Large Leeks (white and light green parts only, chopped)
- 4 sprigs of fresh thyme
- 1 sprig of rosemary
- Bay Leaves
- ½ lemon juice
- salt and pepper to taste

Optional:

chopped fresh chives

1. Add the leeks, chopped onion and garlic in a heating pot with oil. Fry it quickly until it gets soft. Add in the rosemary and thyme

2. Add the cauliflower, broccoli, the chopped potatoes, bay leaves and vegetable stock. Bring to boil and reduce the heat. Cover the pot and cook until the vegetables are soft.

3. Once ready, remove from the heat and take away the bay leaves. Add the coconut milk.

4. With an immersion blender blend the soup until smooth.

5. Add the salt and pepper to taste and the lemon juice. Serve with some more thyme and the fresh chopped chives.

Conclusion:

At first, PCOS can be a really difficult topic to discuss with friends and family. But, what about you? What would you share?

It's quite an intimate topic. I really have difficulty sharing certain matters of privacy even with the closest female members of my family.

Once diagnosed with polycystic ovarian syndrome, it is normal to feel overwhelmed, and so confused to not really understand what to do next. That is being informed about this topic is extremely important. You will feel more confident to talk about it, to share information with the friends or the family members you will be comfortable sharing with. Having them by your side in the fight against PCOS will help you feel more empowered.

PCOS is really about a woman making changes for herself and empowering her to that. I think it is really important to understand what's going on with your body and be able to react and see body and blood tests improvements.

Imagine if a 13 years old girl realizes that the mood swings, the extra pound in the stomach area, the skin problems…are not just the way the things are, but are symptoms. Symptoms of polycystic ovary syndrome are treatable!

I am confident that this book will give you the courage to discuss this subject " more freely". Although it seems like a rare condition, still it can affect a large portion of the female population, so sharing all information is extremely important, as well as connecting and supporting one with another.

Just remember, there is no plan that works for every woman. You will need to find what works best for you and fits into your lifestyle. The right kind of nutrition and lifestyle plan will decrease your symptoms, improve mood and energy levels, help with fertility, aid in weight loss and decrease risk of diabetes and heart disease.

For those living with PCOS, or even diabetes, it can seem overwhelming and takes up a lot of time and mental energy. I always recommend taking small steps when it comes to making changes. Small steps eventually add up to big changes … and improved lifestyle! It's just important to conduct research, be aware of your condition and know where to start! And I deeply hope that this book will motivate you and show how to plan your next steps for a better lifestyle.

And with this, I would consider my mission with this book as accomplished!

P.S. Let me know in the comments which change you started implementing first and how this book helped you! I am really interested to hear about the single experiences. I am reading all comments, and your experience will help the community members as well to feel connected and empowered in their fight with PCOS.

Thank you!
Olivia Stein